PRAISE *for* CUT THROUGH THE NOISE

The importance of this book and its subject cannot be overstated. In my twenty-five years as a wealth strategist, I have assisted families making difficult choices dealing with aging husbands, wives, fathers, and mothers. The stress of disagreement among siblings over the best course of action can tear families apart. *Cut through the Noise* provides authority on how to determine if a facility is right for someone you love, helping to eliminate the guesswork. This book is essential for anyone who has to make decisions about aging loved ones.

I have had the pleasure of knowing Dr. Pobee for the past four years. We have had many conversations about elderly care, since it is close to his heart. His passion and dedication to the aging generation is now being translated into a tool for families in their quest for quality care. With his help, quality care for the elderly will become the norm instead of the exception.

This legacy of love will not only keep families together but will help the next generation (us baby boomers) receive better service and create a better industry.

—James Conaway, LUTCF, CSPG, CRC, **Financial Strategist,**
Co-Owner, Conaway & Conaway
Cohost Smart Money Talk Radio on KCAA 1050AM,
every Monday from 3 pm to 4 pm
www.conawayandconaway.com

The complexities of the nursing-home world can confound and frustrate anyone new to this environment. As a speech pathologist working in long-term care and specifically nursing homes for many years, I can attest to this. *Cut through the Noise* delivers knowledge and insight into the milieu that cares for our elderly, and it will guide you and your loved ones during this vulnerable time.

A Goldsmith, MS CCC-SLP

While *Cut through the Noise* is an invaluable guide for family members and loved ones—particularly adult children directly involved in managing their parents' nursing-home choices and care—this book also goes a long way in expanding the support to adult children who are geographically outside the immediate area. This information is a tool to simplify and enrich communication among adult siblings and other family members through an ever-changing process that is anything but simple or easy. While care-giving responsibilities are rarely evenly divided among family members and friends, educating everyone with an overview of various considerations increases understanding among those having a front-row seat and those whose experience is from afar.

—PAULETTE ENSIGN, PUBLISHER
www.tipsbooklets.com and www.SeniorcareMarketingTools.com

Nursing homes will play a vital role in health care as baby boomers live longer and push the boundaries of the average life expectancy. It will be helpful to educate patients and their family members on what to expect during this important phase of life. They will need to consider all alternatives including skilled-nursing facilities/nursing homes, home health care, retirement centers, and so on. *Cut through the Noise* serves as a great resource in educating patients and their families. It will guide them through the process and eliminate frustrations as they age gracefully.

—VICTOR UGWA, ADMINISTRATOR
Horizon Home Health Agency, Dallas, TX
www.horizonhomehealthagency.com

In my twenty-five-plus years as an administrator, I have held licenses in Missouri, Georgia, Alabama, New Mexico, and currently in Texas. I have experienced a great number of changes to the long-term-care field, both in its delivery and in the funding mechanisms. The demands and expectations from all components continue to be challenging, yet essential. The key leadership teams must continue to find ways to work through the myriad of challenges that lie before us, requiring perseverance, teamwork, and adaptability. Those of us who work "in the trenches" know the confusion and misinformation so many families face. In writing *Cut through the Noise*, I commend Dr. Pobee for taking families by the hand to assist them through the long-term-care journey.

—DOUGLAS A. LINZE, **Licensed Nursing-Facility Administrator**
The Vintage Retirement and Health Care Facility, Denton, TX
www.vintage.seniorcarecentersltc.com

The complexities of long-term care are ever changing. Last year's rules are not the same ones we play by this year. It takes someone who has daily involvement in long-term health care to stay abreast of these changes. So many different regulators and government offices play a role in defining the path of care that they are often at odds with each other. The basic tenant of good long-term care remains unchanged—that is, to give top quality care, the caregiver must love the receiver. But how is it paid for? How do you decide the best location for your loved one? What expectations should you have? I applaud Dr. Pobee's pursuit of these questions and more. He expertly holds your hand through the dynamic process of obtaining the best in long-term care.

—KEVIN NICCUM, **Licensed Nursing-Facility Administrator,**
Executive Director and CEO
Willow Bend Nursing and Rehab
www.willowbendcare.com

The current situation in our health-care system, including long-term care, should not be a surprise to anyone. We have known for years these days would come, and yet we are ill-prepared for the challenge. As a health-care provider and an RN for seventeen years, I can say the insights in this book will help families understand their responsibilities to our seniors as far as concerns ensuring the quality of nursing-home care continues despite the difficult financial times. *Cut through the Noise* is a must-read.

—JEFFREY MERRY, RN
Director of Nursing
Senior Care Beltline, Garland, TX
www.beltline.seniorcarecentersltc.com

Thank goodness for *Cut through the Noise*. Families take heed. This is inside stuff from an insider. I have been a social worker in a long-term-care facility for thirteen years. Caring for the elderly is both challenging and rewarding. The ever-changing Medicare and Medicaid systems often create obstacles in providing quality care to our residents. However, with a dedicated, stable team, a facility can grow and thrive and ultimately achieve the goal of delivering quality and compassionate care to our elderly.

—CASSIE PATTERSON, LBSW
Willow Bend Nursing and Rehab, Mesquite, TX
www.willowbendcare.com

Finally, a comprehensive, insightful book on how to evaluate and maneuver through the maze of long-term and skilled-care options. Dr. Kojo Pobee takes you inside the world where he lives every day. The consummate communicator and educator, his skill and knowledge are unmatched in providing highly skilled medical assessment and ensuring patients' needs are met every day. It is this dedication to long-term care that he has incorporated into this book. As an experienced director of nursing and a published author, I find his writing style concise and easy to read and understand. He addresses multiple aspects of long-term care and encourages readers to determine what is important for their loved one, thus making decisions easier. *Cut through the Noise* is a must-read for all who seek detailed, professional guidance in locating the best facility for any family member.

—Peggy L. Fogle, MS, RN, CHES, QMHP
Pen name: Eliza Beth Rawlins, author of *Dear Douglas*
www.crackedkeyboardproductions.com

CUT THROUGH THE NOISE

CUT THROUGH
THE NOISE

NURSING HOME CARE IN THE BABY BOOMER ERA

A Physician's Advice for Confidently Placing Your Mom,
Dad, Spouse, or Any Senior Family Member

Kojo Pobee, MD, CMD

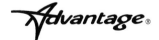

Published by Advantage, Charleston, South Carolina.
Member of Advantage Media Group.

ADVANTAGE is a registered trademark and the Advantage colophon is a trademark of Advantage Media Group, Inc.

Printed in the United States of America.

ISBN: 978-159932-350-3
LCCN: 2013932733

This publication is designed to provide accurate and authoritative information in regard to the subject matter covered. It is sold with the understanding that the publisher is not engaged in rendering legal, accounting, or other professional services. If legal advice or other expert assistance is required, the services of a competent professional person should be sought.

Advantage Media Group is proud to be a part of the Tree Neutral® program. Tree Neutral offsets the number of trees consumed in the production and printing of this book by taking proactive steps such as planting trees in direct proportion to the number of trees used to print books. To learn more about Tree Neutral, please visit www.treeneutral.com. To learn more about Advantage's commitment to being a responsible steward of the environment, please visit www.advantagefamily.com/green

Advantage Media Group is a publisher of business, self-improvement, and professional development books and online learning. We help entrepreneurs, business leaders, and professionals share their Stories, Passion, and Knowledge to help others Learn & Grow™. Do you have a manuscript or book idea that you would like us to consider for publishing? Please visit advantagefamily.com or call 1.866.775.1696.

DEDICATION

To the patients and families I am privileged to care for: this book is for you.

To CNAs, nurses, and all staff members who work in long-term care: You are the unsung heroes who make the system work. Thank you.

To Lawrence LaPalio, MD, my mentor in geriatric medicine: You made geriatrics sexy and dynamic!

To the memory of Danielle Hall of The Health Group,1967-2013, gone so fast, gone so young: You are the standard by which I judge all would-be experts and consultants. Just as you had in all your reports ("Danielle Classics"), I now expect theirs to say, "my analysis is…" and "my recommendation is…"

To the loving memory of Prof. Joseph Orleans Mends Pobee, "The Great": You've been my greatest role model in the practice of medicine, this noblest of professions.

To Dr. Lucy Mary Pobee: Ma, you are a blessing to our family. If JOMP is the head, you are the neck, turning and steering us all in the right direction.

To Joseph Panyin and Joel Kakra, "The Twins," and Caitlyn Emmanuella, "The Girl": I strive to inspire, and I long for each one of you to discover and express your own unique talents and gifts.

To Marian Imelda Pobee, MD, my one and only: Arm-in-arm we tread on our life journey together. You are the best thing that has ever happened to me.

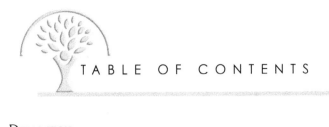

TABLE OF CONTENTS

Kojo Pobee, MD, CMD, is the founder of MD for Seniors, a medical practice dedicated to long-term care that focuses exclusively on delivering physician services to patients where they reside: in nursing homes, assisted living facilities, and occasionally in their homes. In this work, he also collaborates with home-health-care companies and hospice agencies.

Dr. Pobee earned his medical degree in 1988 from the University of Ghana Medical School in Ghana, West Africa. He completed his residency training in internal medicine at the Cook County Hospital in Chicago, Illinois, and his fellowship course in geriatric medicine at the Loyola University Medical Center/Edward Hines Jr. VA Hospital Program, also in Chicago. Board certified in both internal medicine and geriatrics, he has also earned the American Medical Directors Association designation of Certified Medical Director.

Medicine has always been part of the fabric of his life. His late father was a physician; his mother, wife, brother-in-law, a few cousins, and other in-laws are all medical doctors. He says, "If we all got together, we'd have a veritable medical convention!"

PREFACE

Writing this book fulfills the part of my chosen personal mission that reads: "To use my mind, talents, and abilities to be a person of value, rendering useful service to as many people as I can during my lifetime." Most important, this book has the potential to reach a lot more people than my seeing patients one at a time.

My first objective is to raise awareness about the less well-known area of health care called long-term care (LTC). LTC encompasses medical care in skilled-nursing facilities, nursing homes, and assisted-living facilities, as well as services provided by home-health-care companies and hospice agencies.

Second, I want to help seniors and their adult children cut through the negative noise and misinformation about nursing homes. They will come away accurately understanding the potential place of nursing-home care in a person's life cycle.

Third, I want to help families feel in control and to be actively involved in the care and well-being of a loved one, even when that person is in a nursing home. Families still need to participate in decision making at all levels, both medical and nonmedical, as they provide support and comfort to their loved ones.

Finally, I hope you find this book easy and enjoyable to read.

Kojo Pobee, MD, CMD

Dr. Pobee credits Preferred Care with giving the beginning of his nursing-home practice a running start at three of our Dallas-Fort Worth area facilities in 2007. Preferred Care operates more than 100 nursing homes in multiple states.

We like to say the relationship has been mutually beneficial. With the greying of America, Preferred Care and Dr. Pobee's company MD for Seniors have both grown in their related but separate fields over the last few years.

Today, nursing homes are the leading venue for after-hospital care for seniors. This type of facility accounts for more than 50 percent of hospital discharges, including 30 to 40 percent of discharges for rehabilitative care. For many patients recovering from respiratory, cardiac, and neurologic conditions or from surgical procedures, the recuperating process occurs in a skilled-nursing facility/nursing home where patients receive rehabilitation services and nursing care before returning to their own homes or moving to another institution.

The advancing age of the American baby boomer population and the anticipated government health-care policy changes will "push" patients from higher-cost settings such as hospitals to lower-cost arenas such as nursing homes. In fact, the unprecedented growth of the U.S. elderly demographic presents a challenge, not only to the health-care system but also to the families embroiled in the process of "placing" their loved ones in nursing homes.

Are you ready? Probably not.

Post-acute care, long-term care, skilled nursing—these are all grey areas, no pun intended, in most Americans' experience. Dr Pobee's book, *Cut through the Noise*, directed at laymen, does a nice job of demystifying this lesser-known area of health care that is soon to become part of the American psyche.

Devour this book and return to its pages often.

Michael De Cardenas, MD
Corporate Medical Director
Preferred Care Management Group
Plano, TX

INTRODUCTION

On any given day, nearly two million Americans reside in nursing facilities. In the year 2000, approximately 5 percent of all seniors—people aged sixty-five and older—lived in nursing homes. That same year, nearly 20 percent of the oldest of the old (eighty-five and older) could be found in nursing homes. That illustrates one of the major facts about long-term-care medicine—the older a person is, the higher the likelihood of ending up in one of about 16,000 nursing homes in the United States. That's because dependency rises with age due to extensive loss of physical and mental abilities in the later years of life.

Looking ahead as the baby boomer generation ages, one-quarter to one-half of American seniors can expect to be admitted into a nursing home during their lifetimes, either short-term or long-term. Because this is a significant chunk of the population, it means most people will be interacting with a nursing home at some point in their lives—either directly as residents themselves or acting on behalf of a family member.

Living in a nursing home is a situation that many have not yet personally encountered. That's why it's important to dispel the uncertainty and misinformation that prevails. Reading these chapters will help you become a more informed consumer as you assess long-term-care needs for yourself or your loved ones. It opens doors to valuable information that will help you make informed choices now and in the future.

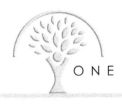

ONE

THE NURSING-
HOME DILEMMA

What do you think of when you hear the term nursing home? Very probably, nothing positive, especially if you've had no experience with these facilities as they exist today.

In a survey published in December 2007 by the Kaiser Public Opinion Spotlight on Long-Term Care, four out of five respondents reported having a personal experience with nursing homes, either as a patient or a visitor. In addition, 68 percent had family members or friends who had been in nursing homes during the preceding three years. But only 35 percent of respondents believed nursing homes were doing a good job. For hospitals, 64 percent said they did a good job, while it was 69 percent for doctors. Nurses rated the highest, with 84 percent of respondents saying they were doing a good job.

For many folks, nursing homes are perceived as being little more than dumping grounds for unwanted elderly people—places of unpleasant odors, wailing, and even death, even places where residents never receive high-quality care.

Why the discrepancy in perception between hospitals and nursing homes? Clinics and big hospitals are familiar to most people and so is the important work carried out within them. That's thanks to the coverage their achievements receive in the popular media.

Unfortunately, nursing homes usually only hit the headlines when something bad happens—e.g., being targeted by fraud investigations, named in personal-injury litigation, or involved in other negative events. Given that this type of story is the only one most people hear, the negative public perception of nursing homes is understandable.

Often, families only consider a nursing-home option when forced by unforeseen health circumstances, such as a family member being discharged after a hospital stay. Typically, people expect their loved one to quickly recover from the illness or injury and then go straight back home.

Many families hear their loved ones adamantly stating, "Promise me you will never, ever put me into a nursing home." Maybe you yourself have said that to your spouse or children. At the time, this may have seemed like a reasonable request, but what happens if one of the family members goes into the hospital? As the discharge date gets closer, it becomes obvious Dad or Mom needs more medical care or hands-on help than can be managed at home. Perhaps your parent needs assistance getting in and out of bed or getting bathed, dressed, fed, and taking medications.

Chances are, you can't be there all the time to assist your parent because you have a job or, for other reasons, you can't safely bring him or her into your home. Events usually happen quickly, taking families by surprise. You may have made that "no nursing home ever" promise to your parent but realize you can't keep it. You feel terribly guilty and the loved one going into the nursing home might feel even worse.

This unhappy series of events happens all the time, as this excerpt from Richard J. Ham and Philip D. Sloane's *Primary Care Geriatrics: A Case-Based Approach* states on p. 676:

Of all the areas of geriatric medicine, nursing homes are maligned and misunderstood the most. The mere mention of nursing homes is often enough to arouse strong negative feelings among patients and physicians alike. These feelings result from incontrovertible facts: nursing homes are institutions; they work with limited resources; and their patients have high levels of disability and generally poor prognoses.

Yet, nursing homes play a vital and well-established role in health care for older persons. For the elderly who cannot find care elsewhere, they provide security, shelter, food, basic care, and a social environment. For the elderly who have been previously isolated, they can open up exciting opportunities in terms of social contact and activities. For families who have struggled with a heavy burden of physical care, nursing homes provide relief, freeing the family's energy to meet the emotional needs of the patient. By managing confused, violent, and dangerous, cognitively impaired patients, nursing homes provide therapy and offer protection to the larger community.

Nursing homes provide a degree of supportive care that is more intensive than rest homes, boarding homes, or most home-care situations, yet far less intensive than the acute-care hospital. They serve a variety of patients, including individuals with acute problems who come for brief rehabilitative stays, persons in the terminal phases of illness, mentally ill persons who no longer require psychiatric hospitalization, and chronically disabled individuals who require daily help with personal care. Nursing homes are modeled after hospitals, with charts, nursing shifts, and institutional routines. Yet the better ones create a homelike feeling, allowing individual freedom of choice to an extent rarely seen in hospitals. The physician's role is less central in the nursing home than in the acute-care hospital, yet active physician involvement is essential to quality nursing-home care.

Many people think of nursing homes as impersonal, yet they can function like valued communities. In these environments, the residents, staff, and professionals who work there spend their lives in close contact with each other. While not everything about any community will be 100 percent positive, on the whole, more good than bad happens in homes like these.

In fact, nursing homes are rapidly improving on many levels—a change driven by the baby boomer consumers who are going into nursing homes themselves or putting their parents in these homes. These consumers are aware, independent-minded, and used to doing their own research online. Clearly, they won't accept a shoddy situation or a bad deal.

RESEARCHING OPTIONS

How do you select the right nursing home for you or your loved one? You can start any online search of nursing homes at www. medicare. gov/nhcompare/. The vast majority of nursing homes in the country have registered at this site, allowing you to review descriptions and assess the quality of the homes listed.

As you may know, everything gets rated these days, including doctors. That means patients and families can become better informed largely because of what is available to them online. Plus people can compare notes about their experiences—something that was more difficult to do before the advent of the Internet.

Thanks to ratings sites and social networking sites, if people own a nursing home or assisted-living facility and want to stay in business, they have to do the right thing by providing a comfortable, clean, safe, and welcoming environment or go out of business. Today, consumers drive the standards more than ever, and if facilities don't keep them up, word gets out quickly.

However, because consumers have a tremendous amount of information available, it can lead to confusion, which is why this book is needed.

NURSING-HOME CARE IS NOT "ONE SIZE FITS ALL"

What is a nursing home? It's a medical facility that houses patients who are unable to care for themselves or are in need of supervised, around-the-clock medical care.

Nursing homes offer the most extensive, highest level of care a person can get outside an acute-care hospital, a long-term acute-care hospital, or an inpatient-rehabilitation hospital. They provide help with personal care such as bathing, dressing, and feeding—all delivered by nurses' aides—as well as skilled nursing care, which includes medical monitoring and treatments performed by nurses. Additional skilled care includes rehabilitation services provided by specially trained professionals such as physical, occupational, and speech therapists. A licensed physician supervises each patient's overall care.

Living in a nursing home also allows patients to be cared for on a continual basis by health-care professionals, including certified nurses' aides, qualified nurses, and trained rehabilitation therapists. In the same vein, nursing homes provide a venue for other long-

term-care (LTC) professionals such as physicians, nurse practitioners, physicians' assistants, psychiatrists, psychologists, podiatrists,
dentists, optometrists, and audiologists to treat patients efficiently.

Overall, patients in nursing homes are safe, cared for, and
monitored better than they could be in their own homes. Most LTC
professionals find a great deal of satisfaction ministering to such a
medically underserved population.

Selecting a facility is much like choosing a college: Some kids
love the big state schools, while others fit into a more intimate
campus and smaller classes. Like colleges, a wide range of nursing-
home models exist, from small and intimate locations to larger communities, each offering a variety of possible experiences.

One way to characterize them is by type of ownership, as the
following chart shows giving approximate proportions of ownership.
(Adapted from Cowles, CM. *Nursing Home Statistical Yearbook*,
2001. Cowles Research Group. Montgomery, MD)

NURSING-HOME OWNERSHIP	PROPORTION
For-Profit	65 percent
Nonprofit	29 percent
Government	6 percent

Currently, 65 percent of nursing homes are privately owned and
for-profit. These homes may be run by big corporations or by small
"mom-and-pop" enterprises.

Nonprofits, including church organizations, operate nearly 30
percent of nursing homes. The U.S. Department of Veterans Affairs

(VA) and other governmental agencies run the remaining 5 percent or so.

Facilities associated with church organizations tend to be open about their religious beliefs and practices, which may or may not fit a potential patient's lifestyle. To qualify for a VA-run place, a patient has to have served in the U.S. armed forces, which makes many people ineligible.

As a rule, the for-profit nursing homes strive to appeal to what the public wants and are the most numerous.

Nursing homes also differ in size, from small to very large. What each person prefers in terms of size depends on individual needs and personality, so it's important to consider questions like "What do I prefer in terms of surrounding activity and population density?" and "Would I like the intimacy of a smaller home better than a larger one?" Take into account that a large facility offers more diversity in personalities as well as more activities and movement, with people in and out of therapy throughout the day.

The following chart (also adapted from Cowles's *Nursing Home Statistical Yearbook*) shows percentages available.

NURSING-FACILITY SIZE	PROPORTION
Fewer than 61 beds	26 percent
61–120 beds	45 percent
More than 120 beds	29 percent

What are some advantages? First, larger facilities have more people residents can interact with. Second, they generally offer more varied opportunities to socialize through scheduled activities.

Managing such numbers of residents can get unwieldy, though, and a shy person might get lost in the crowd.

In addition, staff members at large homes manage a large number of people, so the personal touch may suffer—something that might matter a great deal to you or your loved one. Plus, a bigger facility has to be highly organized, which means it can feel regimented. For instance, moving large numbers of people to the dining hall and back means things have to run strictly on time and happen at a fast pace. Some people like that; in fact, some may *need* that because they get bored otherwise.

Take time to compare the types of atmosphere you'd find at a bigger facility versus a smaller one. What suits you or your loved one best?

WHO LIVES IN NURSING HOMES?

The range of answers may surprise you. The following examples are real residents, although their identities have been changed to preserve their privacy.

J. S. is a sixty-year-old man undergoing rehabilitation therapy after a planned total knee replacement.

M. Z. is a ninety-year-old woman recovering from severe pneumonia and still receiving intravenous antibiotics.

M. J. is a seventy-two-year-old man with terminal metastatic lung cancer and on hospice care.

A. J. is a thirty-year-old male who was in a car accident; he has traumatic brain injury (mental impairment), quadriplegia (paralysis of all four of his limbs), a neurogenic bladder, and a neurogenic bowel (impaired nerve control of bladder and bowel that affects functioning).

S. Q. is a twenty-five-year-old man with cerebral palsy (muscle paralysis present at birth), multiple contractures (drawn up limbs), and a gastrostomy tube for tube feeding (an opening created in the stomach with a feeding tube passed into it to transport liquid nutrition feedings).

H. A. is a twenty-five-year old woman with multiple sclerosis, difficulty walking, and impaired activities of daily living (impaired personal self-care and mobility).

R. M. is a forty-year-old woman who is morbidly obese (she weighs 450 pounds); she is unable to walk and care for herself.

D. N. is a forty-six-year-old diabetic with a history of multiple heart attacks and an amputation of the right leg below the knee. He receives hemodialysis for end-stage renal failure.

S. J. is a seventy-year-old woman with severe dementia from Alzheimer's disease who is dependent in all of her activities of daily living (ADLs).

C. S. is a sixty-five-year-old man with a history of stroke and vascular dementia.

A. H. is a forty-year-old man with mental retardation who is pleasant and friendly but unable to manage his intellectual/instrumental activities of daily living (IADLs). He has no siblings, and his parents are too old to take care of him.

J. D. is a thirty-year-old woman with bipolar disorder (a psychiatric disorder) who is unable to manage her IADLs and has no family support.

Some long-term residents live permanently in nursing homes; some short-term residents go to nursing homes between their hospital stay and ultimately return home. This usually happens after an illness or major surgery and is regarded as a bump in the road rather than a lifestyle change. However, as they get older and more infirm, they may have to return to the nursing home. At that point, the stay may be permanent.

In nursing homes, the two populations, short-term and long-term, coexist. When most people talk about nursing homes though, they tend only to think about the geriatric population that do, in fact, form the majority of residents. Indeed, the baby boomer generation is driving the growth of those numbers.

However, a younger group of people is entering nursing homes at earlier ages than before and in increasing numbers. They're being placed in nursing homes because of two epidemics: diabetes and obesity.

If you developed diabetes at twenty-five years of age or earlier and your condition has been difficult to control, you can expect that, in the ensuing ten to twenty years, you may have diabetes-related complications. These complications include heart attacks, congestive heart failure, strokes, kidney failure, visual impairment from eye retinopathy, or limb amputations. Worst case, you could have several complications, be debilitated, on dialysis, and even completely blind.

Sadly, people in their early to mid-forties are experiencing these complications. Where do these relatively young yet seriously disabled people go for care? If they don't have family members who can care for them at home, they end up in a nursing home. As a group, they're a significant growing portion of the nursing-home population.

A similar trend is happening among people who are morbidly overweight. Complications of this condition include diabetes, hypertension, coronary heart disease, obstructive sleep apnea, cancer, gout, and disabling arthritis. Imagine being so obese, you can't move much less care for yourself.

An increasing number of younger people find themselves in this situation. In fact, some nursing homes actually cater to this niche. If an obese person goes to a hospital and can't immediately go home for medical reasons, then he or she goes into a nursing home to recuperate and possibly reside there long term.

In addition to the elderly, young patients with diabetic complications, and the young obese, other residents include people who've had catastrophic accidents with permanent injuries and patients with psychiatric diagnoses who can't function in society on their own. They also make up part of the nursing-home population.

WHAT IS YOUR NOTION OF NURSING HOMES?

Given the aging baby boomer generation, their elderly parents, those with lifestyle-related medical conditions, catastrophic accidents, and mental illness, increasingly more people will have contact with nursing homes in the years to come. Does that notion send chills down your spine? Perhaps your conception of nursing homes is anything but comforting. You might even regard being in nursing homes as heartbreaking.

Heartbreaking is a strong word. And hearing what misinformed people think about nursing homes can be disturbing to dedicated LTC workers. Indeed, most professionals who work every day in long-term care could be called "bullish" on nursing homes, that is, they have positive opinions and hold a highly optimistic point of view about them.

After all, nursing homes provide much-needed structure and important socializing to their residents who might otherwise be overwhelmed, lonely, or marginalized. These homes bring groups of people together. Within each one is a team working for the residents' well-being, meeting their housing and feeding needs as well as their need for social interaction. It happens because the home has an organized system that helps its employees see to all that. This point emphasizes the importance of this book, *Cut through the Noise,* because it dispels the myths about nursing homes and the care received there, and it helps consumers know what to look for when the need arises.

The United States is fortunate in having a robust nursing-home industry. In many other parts of the world, extended family members have to pitch in and care for their elderly or infirm. Nieces and nephews, not only daughters and sons, get involved.

But because of the American lifestyle in which families are so mobile and often live far apart, many young relatives can't easily look after older family members. Nursing homes provide the solution so that vulnerable people aren't left alone in their homes to waste away.

Chapter Six addresses the guilt factor, which is a common reaction to putting a family member into a nursing home. Please don't buy into that notion. You can overcome that by placing your loved one in a secure place and then making sure they get the care they need. That requires visiting your loved one often, interacting with the staff, and ensuring that they are being attended to.

Remember, your loved one can likely come to your home for weekends, or go out for lunch and shopping sprees. Gradually, the facility becomes, in a very real sense, your loved one's home: A home with extra benefits where each person receives needed services.

Again, being placed in a nursing home may not be ideal for your family, but it may be the best solution for a given situation. It may simply be the right thing to do.

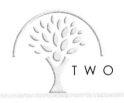

THE LONG-TERM-CARE CONTINUUM

In our overstretched society in which many dual-income families deal with multiple responsibilities, the old model of caring for disabled or ill parents at home doesn't work in the long run.

In America today, if adult children do bring a parent into their home, typically they don't receive much support from siblings or other extended family members spread out across this vast country. Often, one of the adult children winds up shouldering the bulk of the burden, all the while raising his or her own children. Many baby boomers find themselves in a "sandwich generation" situation. On the one hand, they have to deal with caring for an aging parent; on the other hand, they still have to raise their children and manage their own lives. As their responsibilities increase dramatically, they feel squeezed.

In the 21st century, most Americans don't live in communal groupings. This dynamic has fostered the creation of—and continues to sustain—the nursing-home industry. American culture or society is simply not ready or able to handle the elderly within its communities.

Naturally, most seniors prefer to age *in place*—that is, to live out their years in their own homes and communities. In reality, as people get older, they experience extensive loss of functional abilities, which can compromise their health and safety. Chapter Three addresses this functional ability, how it's measured, and how losing it plays into the decision to place individuals into long-term-care facilities.

CARE FOR BABY BOOMERS

The first of the baby boomers—the generation born between 1946 and 1964—turned sixty-five in 2011. In 2010, the census counted 40.3 million elderly aged sixty-five and over in the United States, making up 13 percent of the population.

Because of its large numbers, this generation will require more long-term-care facilities than ever before. By 2030, the elderly will form 22 percent of the U.S. population, up from 13 percent in 2010. The expected 9 to 10 percent increase of over-sixty-fives is being experienced right now.

In 2009, more than 90 percent of America's elderly were living independently in the community; nearly 4 percent lived in nursing homes (1.3 million), and almost 3 percent lived in assisted living facilities (900,000). These percentages of people needing long-term care may not sound like a lot, but if you consider actual numbers—and they're on the increase—then each percentage point becomes significant.

What exactly is *long-term care* or LTC—terms that will become commonplace as this aging population grows?

LTC refers to a spectrum of health, social, and personal-care services provided to the disabled or chronically ill of any age. This type of care is given over an extended time in a variety of settings.

Long-term care actually evolved from the welfare system, not the health-care world. That partly explains why it has an understated presence in the health-care system. It also explains why LTC includes substantial social and psychiatric services in addition to medical health services.

THE DEPENDENCY PATHWAY

What types of long-term-care settings exist? Think of them in categories depending on the level of care needed. To place these levels into context, consider the idea of the *dependency pathway*. This pathway from A to I categorizes people from the most independent to the most infirm and shows where they reside.

A. Independent elderly living in their personal homes and apartments

B. Independent elderly living in senior communities

C. People living in rest homes (group homes)

D. Residents in assisted living facilities and memory-care centers

E. Residents in nursing homes

F. Patients in freestanding rehabilitation hospitals

G. Patients in long-term acute-care hospitals

H. Patients on admission in acute-care hospitals

I. Patients in ICUs and CCUs within acute-care hospitals

Within this dependency pathway, the long-term-care settings are C, D, and E—namely, rest homes (group homes), assisted-living facilities/memory-care centers, and nursing homes.

Additional services supporting the aging population include senior centers, adult day-care centers, and adult day health-care centers. These are facility-based LTC settings that don't provide room or board.

Home-health and hospice agencies provide services to residents in many of these LTC settings. They are not mentioned in the list, but a very small number of freestanding, hospice inpatient facilities also exist.

The following chart summarizes options on the pathway:

LONG-TERM-CARE SERVICE	EXAMPLES
Facility-based, without room and board	Senior centers Adult day-care centers Adult day health-care centers
Facility-based, with room and board	Rest homes (group homes) Assisted-living facilities Memory-care centers Nursing homes Freestanding inpatient hospice facilities
Nonfacility-based	Home-health agencies Hospice agencies

A *senior center* is a place where independent-living, cognitively intact healthy seniors can go to socialize. Senior centers provide meals and social activities but not organized health services. These centers receive some government funding.

Next are *adult day-care centers* and *adult day health-care centers*, usually combined in one facility. The adult day-care part provides meals, activities, and some supervision by professional staff. Certain people need the supervision in this setting because of their cognitive impairment. This is the type of place to which community-dwelling seniors with dementia can be taken to spend time safely and enjoy social interaction and stimulation.

An extension of adult day-care centers, *adult day health-care facilities* provide medical and nursing care, along with nutritional supplements (such as Boost and Ensure) to augment their food intake. Doctors may make rounds in these facilities; some centers make rehabilitation therapy available. Overall, they cater to individuals who aren't totally incapacitated and still live in the community. Their family members can't be there for them during the day, usually because of work schedules. In effect, these facilities chaperone seniors in the family members' absence, giving them a safe place to remain, while providing some health-care services.

On the next level are *rest homes* (group homes) and *assisted-living facilities*, which are residential options. The physical establishments can range from single-family homes to large buildings. These settings, considered social rather than medical venues, aren't regulated as strictly as nursing homes, which are medical venues.

Assisted-living facilities typically provide three meals a day and housekeeping service. They have 24-hour security and help residents with their activities of daily living. (Chapter Four delves into more about personal-care activities such as bathing, feeding, dressing, and so forth.) At assisted-living facilities, some residents are reminded to take their medicines; others have theirs administered by the staff. Transportation may be provided.

Some assisted-living facilities have memory-care units within them, but there are also freestanding *memory-care centers* that focus only on people who have various kinds of dementia. Both have staff members who are specially trained to deal with dementia patients. The centers are designed to mitigate safety concerns for patients who are apt to wander.

Nursing homes accommodate those who are too infirm or ill for the less comprehensive care available in assisted-living facilities. Nursing homes are medical facilities that operate within strict state and federal guidelines. Patients are admitted either for a short stay or a long stay. "Short stay" means six months or less, while "long-term/permanent" means more than six months.

The table that follows illustrates the different categories of nursing-home residents.

TYPE OF NURSING-HOME RESIDENT	EXAMPLES
SHORT-TERM (days to six months)	
(i) Short-term rehabilitation ("Rehab-to-home")	After hip fracture repairs and hip or knee replacements; after strokes
(ii) Subacute (medically unstable)	Recovering from infections (PNA, UTI); poorly controlled diabetes mellitus; cardiovascular/pulmonary disease (CHF, COPD)
(iii) Terminally ill	End-stage cancer End-stage dementia
LONG-TERM (greater than six months)	
(i) Primarily cognitively impaired	Dementia; psychiatric problems
(ii) Primarily physically impaired	Musculoskeletal, neurologic, cardiac, or pulmonary disease (also includes younger patients with diabetic complications, obesity complications, and paraplegics/quadriplegics)

| (iii) Both cognitively and physically impaired | Dementia plus musculoskeletal, neurologic, cardiac, or pulmonary disease (also includes younger patients with traumatic brain injury) |

Table adapted from Ouslander, J.G. et. al. Annals of Internal Medicine 1994;120:584-592

SHORT-TERM CARE OPTIONS

After orthopedic surgery (or any other surgery whether elective or an emergency), elderly patients need to get back on their feet before going home. The nursing home is one setting where rehab therapy can be done during a relatively short stay.

Similarly, some seniors come out of the hospital after being admitted for pneumonia or decompensated congestive heart failure and are too weak or debilitated to go home. Both kinds of deconditioned patient need skilled nursing in addition to rehab. In the surgery cases, some patients may need wound care for their incisions. In turn, those who are medically unstable often need to continue receiving complex medication regimens, such as intravenous antibiotics, respiratory inhalation treatments, or tube feeding.

Finally, the *terminally ill* hospice patients are classified as "short stay" because they're not expected to live beyond six months. Toward the end of life, their care needs may be too much for their caregivers to handle at home, even with in-home hospice help. As a result, they are admitted to nursing homes where they receive collaborative care from both nursing-facility staff and hospice workers.

NURSING HOMES AS AN LTC OPTION

Long-term-care patients—those who remain in nursing homes from six months to several years—fall into one of three groups:

- cognitively impaired
- physically impaired
- cognitively and physically impaired

Patients typically end up in nursing homes permanently if they fail rehab, or if they are admitted with the intent of remaining there right from the start.

In all cases, permanent placement usually means there isn't enough family support to manage the patients' activities of daily living at home. Psychiatric patients are admitted for permanent residence only when they aren't a danger to themselves or to others. Unstable and psychotic patients are stabilized in acute-care hospitals or psychiatric hospitals before they can be considered acceptable for nursing-home placement.

The nomenclature of nursing homes can be confusing. It's best to think of each nursing home as a combination of skilled-nursing facility and nursing facility (SNF/NF). What are these?

- SNFs are short-term, skilled-nursing/rehab beds (Medicare beds plus Managed Medicare beds plus commercial insurance beds).
- NFs are long-term, permanent beds (Medicaid/custodial beds plus private pay beds).

The nursing-facility (NF) part is comprised of nonskilled beds, certified as such by each state's nursing home licensing department, and labeled *Medicaid beds*. They are called *Medicaid beds* because Medicaid is the main payor for nonskilled stays in nursing homes. Some of the nonskilled beds may be ear-marked for private pay (PP) residents.

The skilled-nursing-facility (SNF) part consists of skilled beds certified by the same state licensing department and called *Medicare beds*. They are called *Medicare beds* because Medicare funds most skilled nursing home stays. Some of the skilled beds are earmarked for Managed Medicare patients and the commercially insured. The skilled beds are used for short-term rehab patients, while the Medicaid and private-pay beds are used for long-term residents.

Private-pay rooms or beds shouldn't be confused with private rooms. Private-pay rooms/beds are reserved for long-term residents who have the funds to pay out of pocket for their room and board. Private rooms are single-occupant rooms with a skilled-nursing/rehab bed for patients who request that privilege. Sometimes, all the bed types (skilled and nonskilled) are intermingled. However, increasingly more facilities are grouping the skilled beds in existing wings or in newly built wings with rehab therapy gyms incorporated.

The *nursing-home item* completes the category of facility-based long-term care services. In a category of their own, *home-health-care companies* and *hospice agencies* provide nonfacility, community-based long-term care services. Hospices can service residents in private homes, rest homes, assisted-living facilities, and nursing homes. Home health agencies can do the same except for nursing home residents.

As workers of home health and hospice agencies, nurses' aides provide personal care, assisting with the activities of daily living, such as transferring, toileting, bathing, dressing, and feeding. The Joint Commission on Accreditation of Healthcare Organizations (JCAHO) defines *home health* care as follows:

> *Home health services involve the provision of any health care services by health care professionals to a patient in his or her place of residence. These services include, but are not limited*

to, performance assessments; provision of care, treatment, or counseling; and/or monitoring of the patient's health status by nurses (both intermittent skilled and private duty), occupational therapists, physical therapists, speech-language pathologists, audiologists, social workers, dieticians, dentists, physicians, and other licensed health care professionals in the patient's home. It also includes the extension or follow-up of health care services provided by hospital professional staff in the patient's home.

The use of the home-health-care option is increasing because many believe it's a cost-effective, alternative means of delivering health care to those who meet the criteria.

Hospice agencies provide end-of-life care for terminally ill people who, by definition, are not expected to live for more than six months. JCAHO defines *hospice* as follows:

Hospice is an organized program that consists of services provided and coordinated by an interdisciplinary team to meet the needs of a patient who is diagnosed with a terminal illness and has a limited life span. The program specializes in palliative management of pain and other physical symptoms, meeting the psychosocial and spiritual needs of the patient and the patient's family, use of volunteers, and provision of bereavement care to survivors. Hospice includes, but is not limited to, all programs licensed as hospices and Medicare-certified hospice programs. All services provided by the hospice (for example, pharmacy, home medical equipment services) and care provided in all settings (for example, inpatient, nursing home) are included.

Hospice care workers assist people to die with dignity while helping families deal with loss. They have special skills and training to support patients as they move toward the end of life.

The phrase long-term care (LTC) covers a variety of services provided in physical settings and a number of nonfacility services available in the community. The facility or service that you, your spouse, or your parent qualifies for depends on specific needs and the amount of care required.

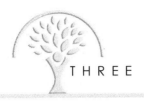

THREE

WHEN IS IT TIME TO CONSIDER NURSING-HOME CARE?

Usually, a dramatic event, illness, or injury sends someone into an acute-care hospital and then on to a nursing home to recuperate. Initially, loved ones assume the patient will only be in the hospital for a short time and then go back home to normal living. Because most cases of nursing-home placement result from a sudden event, careful planning usually doesn't happen. In fact, only a small percentage of residents find placement in the appropriate long-term-care setting after receiving deliberate outpatient consultation and evaluation by trained medical personnel.

In discussing who needs nursing-home care, it's important to understand how physicians—and geriatricians in particular—conclude which setting best serves a patient. The usual medical examination focuses on the person's nervous system, cardiac, respiratory, abdominal, and so on. While this provides a great deal of information about physical systems, it doesn't give much information about the patient's functional abilities. For instance, a neurological examination will tell a physician a great deal about a patient's muscle strength and reflexes, but it may not indicate if the patient is continent or can walk independently, transfer unassisted, and get dressed alone.

The ejection fraction of a patient with heart failure, the FEV1 of someone with COPD, the hemoglobin A1c of a diabetic, and the MRI of a stroke patient all provide data that physicians use to manage these conditions. However, none of that technical information describes how a patient is actually getting on in real-world situations.

Because the usual medical examinations performed on patients do not adequately evaluate function, geriatricians use a variety of standardized tools and techniques to assess function. Specifically, they assess each patient's combination of medical illnesses, physical impairments, and social supports to see how the person performs at home and in the community. Can heart-failure patients with mild dementia manage their own medication regimens? Can patients who have had small strokes safely get to and from restrooms? Can partially blind diabetics who live alone draw up and give themselves insulin injections?

The gold standard in geriatric medicine for determining a patient's overall status is the *geriatric functional screening assessment.* This evaluation includes an assessment of two kinds of Activities of Daily Living, ADLs and IADLs, as well as vision, hearing, mobility, cognition, social supports, continence, depression, medication use, and nutrition, thereby providing a thorough overview of the whole person.

Unfortunately, as of 2008, there are only about 7,100 doctors board-certified in geriatrics in the U.S. Geriatric training only recently became a regular part of medical-school curricula. Thankfully, through continuing medical education courses, practicing internal medicine and family medicine doctors are learning to apply functional screening tools. Also, people can turn to geriatric-care planners to facilitate the whole assessment and placement process.

Another option is to get spouses, adult children, and other care-givers to proactively take control and feel empowered to help. Family members *themselves* can periodically fill out the ADL and IADL instruments and, based on the results they obtain, assess if they should seek expert help in getting a full-scale functional evaluation.

START WITH ADLS

There are two groups of ADL: the basic/essential/physical activities of daily living, or ADLs, and the instrumental/intellectual activities of daily living, called IADLs. The Katz Index (for ADLs) and the Lawton-Brody Scale (for IADLs) are tables clinicians use in actual practice to perform these assessments. These diagrams show the components of ADLs and IADLs along with what the scores indicate. Both are simple enough for laymen to use, score, and interpret easily.

Adaptations of these forms follow.

Katz Index of Independence in Activities of Daily Living

ACTIVITIES Points (1 or 0)	INDEPENDENCE (1 point) NO supervision, direction or personal assistance.	DEPENDENCE (0 points) WITH supervision, direction, personal assistance or total care.
BATHING Points: _____	(1 POINT) Bathes self completely or needs help in bathing only a single part of the body such as the back, genital area or disabled extremity.	(0 POINTS) Need help with bathing more than one part of the body, getting in or out of the tub or shower. Requires total bathing.
DRESSING Points: _____	(1 POINT) Get clothes from closets and drawers and puts on clothes and outer garments complete with fasteners. May have help tying shoes.	(0 POINTS) Needs help with dressing self or needs to be completely dressed.
TOILETING Points: _____	(1 POINT) Goes to toilet, gets on and off, arranges clothes, cleans genital area without help.	(0 POINTS) Needs help transferring to the toilet, cleaning self or uses bedpan or commode.
TRANSFERRING Points: _____	(1 POINT) Moves in and out of bed or chair unassisted. Mechanical transfer aids are acceptable.	(0 POINTS) Needs help in moving from bed to chair or requires a complete transfer.
CONTINENCE Points: _____	(1 POINT) Exercises complete self control over urination and defacation.	(0 POINTS) Is partially or totally incontinent of bowel or bladder.
FEEDING Points: _____	(1 POINT) Gets food from plate into mouth without help. Preparation of food may be done by another person.	(0 POINTS) Needs partial or total help with feeding or requires parenteral feeding.

Total Points: _____

Score of 6 = High, patient is independent.

Score of 0 = Low, patient is very dependent.

**Slightly adapted. Katz S., Down, TD, Cash, HR, et al. (1970) progress in the development of the index of ADL. Gerontologist 10:20-30. Copyright The Gerontological Society of America.
Reproduced by permission of the publisher.

Instrumental Activities of Daily Living Scale (IADL)

A. Ability to use telephone

1. Operates telephone on own initiative: looks up and dials numbers, etc. — 1
2. Dials a few well-known numbers — 1
3. Answers telephone but does not dial — 1
4. Does not use telephone at all — 0

B. Shopping

1. Takes care of all shopping needs independently — 1
2. Shops independently for small purchases — 0
3. Needs to be accompanied on any shopping trip — 0
4. Completely unable to shop — 0

C. Food Preparation

1. Plans, prepares and serves adequate meals independently — 1
2. Prepares adequate meals if supplied with ingredients — 0
3. Heats, serves and prepares meals or prepares meals but does not maintain adequate diet — 0
4. Needs to have meals prepared and served — 0

D. Housekeeping

1. Maintains house alone or with occasional assistance (e.g. "heavy work domestic help") — 1
2. Performs light daily tasks such as dishwashing, bed making — 1
3. Performs light daily tasks but cannot maintain acceptable level of cleanliness — 1
4. Needs help with all home maintenance tasks — 1
5. Does not participate in any housekeeping tasks — 0

E. Laundry

1. Does personal laundry completely — 1
2. Launders small items: rinses stockings, etc. — 1
3. All laundry must be done by others — 0

F. Mode of Transportation

1. Travels independently on public transportation or drives own car — 1
2. Arranges own travel via taxi, but does not otherwise use public transportation — 1
3. Travels on public transportation when accompanied by another — 1
4. Travel limited to taxi or automobile with assitance of another — 0
5. Does not travel at all — 0

G. Responsibility for own medications

1. Is responsible for taking medication in correct dosages at correct time — 1
2. Takes responsiblity if medication is prepared in advance in separate dosage — 0
3. Is not capable of dispensing own medication — 0

H. Ability to Handle Finances

1. Manages financial matters independently (budgets, writes checks, pays rent, bills, goes to bank), collects and keeps track of income — 1
2. Manages day-to-day purchases, but needs help with banking, major purchases, etc. — 1
3. Incapable of handling money — 0

For women score on all 8 Domains: Summary score ranges from 0 (low function, dependent) to 8 (high function, independent).

For men score on 5 Domains: historically, food preparation, housekeeping and laundering have been excluded.

In general, scoring is better used to track change in an individual over time, rather than to compare different people.

Source: Lawton, M.P., and Brody, E.M. "Assessment of older people: Self-maintaining and instrumental activities of daily living." Gerontologist 9:179-186, (1969).

Copyright (c) The Gerontological Society of America. Used by permission of the Publisher.

SCORING

Use these ADL and IADL tools to assess the scores of a family member who may need some of the long-term-care services discussed in Chapter 2, perhaps even nursing home care. For the ADL scale, the summary score ranges from 0 (low-functioning, dependent) to 6 (high-functioning, independent). With the IADL scale, women score in all eight domains, with the summary score ranging from 0 (low-functioning, dependent) to 8 (high-functioning, independent). Men, on the other hand, score in only five domains, with food preparation, housekeeping, and laundering not being male duties, historically. If your male family member does perform these tasks, include them in the scoring.

Compare the scores. In both cases, the lower the score the more dependent or the more help the individual needs with those tasks. Simplistically speaking, the IADLs are tasks that, if needed, can be performed on an individual's behalf by family or community resources. The ADL tasks can also be done for an individual, but these activities are more physical and labor intensive than IADL tasks.

Keep in mind the *degree* of dependency. A family member can be dependent in terms of IADLs but independent in terms of ADLs. With good family or community support, such a person might be able to live in his or her own home. Without the family/community support, a rest home or an assisted-living facility could be considered. If the impaired IADLs are largely due to cognitive limitations such as dementia, moving into a memory-care center might be appropriate.

If your family member is highly dependent in terms of the more-physical ADLs, the logistics of keeping him or her at home become complicated and a nursing home may be the only option. Having to manage bladder or bowel incontinence in particular is often the final straw that precipitates a nursing-home placement.

Armed with basic ADL and IADL information, you can get an idea of how doctors will view your loved one's situation. Use this data to determine if you can bring in the support your loved one requires (through family members, friends, and church members, and by tapping into any other community). At this time, you can gauge if your loved one needs services that an adult day-care center or home-health agency could provide. Perhaps seek the help of a geriatric-care planner.

PROFILE OF THE TYPICAL NURSING-HOME RESIDENT

Although there's an increasing number of residents under sixty-five years old due to (1) the diabetes-obesity epidemics/complications, and (2) neurological/catastrophic/psychiatric patients, that population (as of 2009) was only 14.2 percent. The majority of nursing-home residents fall into the following description.

- A typical resident is a widowed, separated, or divorced woman in her mid-eighties who shows mild forms of memory loss and dementia.
- She was most recently in a hospital before entering a nursing home. The leading admission diagnosis for nursing-home residents is heart disease followed by mental disorders and injuries.
- Although she may be physically healthy for her age, she needs help with about four of the five ADLs (eating, dressing, bathing, transferring and mobility, and toileting).
- She has three to five medical diagnoses. She takes nine medications—6.7 routine prescription medications per day and 2.7 additional medications on an as-needed basis.

- Cognitive impairments and mental disorders are the most common conditions in nursing-home residents.
- The most commonly prescribed medications are gastrointestinal agents (including laxatives, enemas, and acid secretion reducers), analgesics (including acetaminophen and aspirin), cardiovascular medications (including Digoxin, diuretics, and nitrates), vitamins and supplements (including multivitamins and potassium), and psychoactive medications (including sedatives and hypnotics, antipsychotics, and antidepressants).

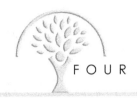

SHOPPING FOR A NURSING HOME

Once you've decided—for yourself or on behalf of a loved one—to make the move to a nursing home (or circumstances have made the decision for you), how do you choose the best one?

In most cases, something forces the decision. Often, it's a hospitalization due to a sudden illness when the patient is too weak to go home. Even if family support at home exists, the patient may need to finish off IV antibiotics or other treatments in a supervised manner. Perhaps the doctor has ordered a course of rehabilitation therapy.

At that point, hospital staff members recommend a nursing-home stay so your loved one can receive these services. Chances are, you will receive guidance from case managers and discharge planners in this situation.

Another less urgent scenario occurs when a family member resides in an assisted-living facility but experiences declining health or functional status. Even with what's available in an assisted-living facility, it simply may not have enough resources for the care your loved one needs. Similar to the hospital situation, in an assisted-living facility, your family could receive help from its social worker in finding a nursing home.

In yet another situation, your loved one might go straight from home in the community into a nursing facility on the recommendation of a primary-care doctor or geriatric specialist. There too, someone in the doctor's office will help coordinate the transition. In all of these situations, help is available to get a short list of suitable nursing homes.

However, it is possible you might have to start the search from scratch on your own if, for instance, the doctor's office doesn't have the staff capability to assist you that way. Even then, you can likely find geriatric care managers/planners in the community who can be hired for a fee. (Use an online search engine such as Google under the term "geriatric care managers" or something similar.)

When shopping for a nursing home, begin by talking to your family, friends, neighbors, coworkers, and church members. They can often offer you recommendations, especially about places near you. They may have had experiences, good or bad, with local nursing homes so their personal opinions can be extremely helpful.

Keep in mind you want a nursing home close to the people who will visit the patient most often, not necessarily a facility in the patient's own neighborhood. It's not unheard of to relocate to another state if that's where most of a person's family resides. For example, if the patient is living alone in Texas with no family close by, that loved one may have to relocate to Connecticut to be placed in a facility where family can visit easily and often.

After determining a location, next consider if there are any special benefits due to the patient. For example, military veterans and some of their family members may have VA benefits that cover the costs of nursing home care. Perhaps the person might benefit from being close to communities where he or she has religious affiliations that would provide support.

Consider any health services your loved one may need, especially coming out of an acute-care hospital situation. For example, your family member might still need IV fluids or IV antibiotics. If the patient has a tracheotomy and needs to be on a ventilator, find a facility that handles that level of care. Remember, not all facilities are equipped or staffed to provide all services.

In addition, find out about the facility's rehabilitation services. What staff and gym facilities do they have? What equipment does the gym have? What experience does the staff have?

Be sure to note how many beds are in the facility; this is how a facility's size is measured. Size is a personal preference, so ask yourself if your family member will adapt more easily to a large place or a small, homelike atmosphere? It simply depends on what he or she is comfortable with.

If your loved one has dementia, that is a significant factor in your choice. Elopement or wandering from the facility is a major concern with dementia, so find a place that has a *secure unit* or provides other safety features. Some memory-care facilities specialize in patients who have dementia, but they are assisted-living facilities, not nursing homes, so they may not be equipped to handle other medical issues pertinent to your family member. Many nursing homes can and do accept patients suffering from dementia, so ask specifically about their dementia unit or how they otherwise manage dementia residents.

Look at the residents' rooms and ask about all the options available. There may be single rooms, rooms with two beds, even rooms with three or four beds. What you choose will depend on personal preference as well as your funding resources.

Also consider the facility's smoking and pet policies. Whether your family member smokes or has a pet or not, ask how the facility deals with these issues.

GOVERNMENT RESOURCES AS A START

To start your research, you can turn to the government for basic information on nursing homes. The Centers for Medicare & Medicaid Services (CMS)—the government agency that oversees the Medicare and Medicaid programs—offers four publications you can access from the Internet. You can also request free copies to be mailed to you by calling 1-800-MEDICARE (1-800-633-4227).

The four resource publications are described here:

- *Medicare Coverage of Skilled-Nursing-Facility Care* contains detailed information about Medicare-covered skilled care, including your rights and protections and where to get help with questions.
- *Your Guide to Choosing a Nursing Home* contains useful tips about choosing a facility and includes a nursing-home tour checklist.
- *The Medicare and You Handbook* presents a summary of Medicare benefits, rights, and protections; it also includes answers to the most frequently asked questions about Medicare.
- *Medicare's Nursing Home Compare* provides a summary of the information found on the Nursing Home Compare website.

You can discover detailed information using the Nursing Home Compare tool at http://www.medicare.gov/NHCompare. On this site, you can search by zip code and find nursing homes in your area as well as the size of each facility (in terms of number of beds) and also the number of Medicare versus Medicaid beds at each facility. If the facility has any special medical services available (e.g., ventilators, wound care), you'll find them listed on the site as well. You can also find information about the facility's ownership, such as whether it is a for-profit, nonprofit, or government-run organization.

Using this site, you can compare nursing facilities according to the Nursing Home Compare five-star quality rating, health inspections, staffing, quality measures, and fire-safety inspections. The five-star quality rating system (the most commonly used of these five measures) gives site visitors an overall score of nursing homes. You can read about meaningful differences between high-performing and low-performing facilities, plus it has easy-to-use information to help you make choices and data to use when talking to nursing-home staff about the quality of care.

If a facility has earned one or two stars while others have four or five, you may want to save time by making an initial choice based on that rating. However, if events are happening quickly, you likely won't be able to do this research in a leisurely manner. You might have to rush through all the elements of the decision-making process, including site visits. If you have early indications that things aren't going well and this might be a viable option down the road, do the legwork now. This can save you and your family time and trouble in case the need to find a nursing home suddenly becomes acute.

PERSONAL SITE VISITS

Suppose you've taken the advice of your doctor, social worker, friends, or neighbors, and have a short list of facilities based on what's available and your current needs. You're ready to start the process of personal site visits. Start by telephoning each of the nursing homes on your list and ask for an appointment to take a facility tour. In most cases, the person you are looking to place won't be able to come with you on this initial tour because of physical or mental impairments.

It's best not to show up at a facility on an initial visit and demand an impromptu tour. Instead, be sure someone is available to show you around and answer your questions.

Go to your appointment ready to take notes. In Chapter Five and on the Nursing Home Compare site, you'll find a comprehensive nursing-home tour checklist you can print out and take with you. Augment it with your own observations as you go along. Do *not* depend on memory or you will get confused. Multiple nursing-home visits tend to run together when you reflect on them.

Chapter Five discusses exactly what you should pay attention to on those initial visits.

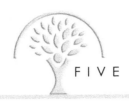

WHAT TO LOOK FOR IN A NURSING-HOME VISIT

Ultimately, no research can tell you more about a nursing home's appropriateness for your loved one than what you can discover by visiting it yourself. *A site visit is a must.* If you can't do it yourself, ask someone whose judgment you trust to do it for you. Do not skip, for any reason, this essential first step in making your choice.

Ideally, you'll visit the most promising facilities more than once. Going on different days and at different times of day gives you a truer picture—more than a snapshot—of what life is like there. However, to accommodate on-site research, be sure to narrow down your choices to a manageable number before you begin the visiting process. By narrowing your list to three to five places, you are less likely to become overwhelmed.

Your subsequent visits can be unannounced, but that first visit should be by appointment. When you arrive, take time to connect with somebody knowledgeable who can show you around and give you an official tour. Expect your guide to be welcoming and happy to show you around. Ideally, also meet the facility administrator and the director of nursing. Their combined input should answer all your questions about both administrative and clinical matters.

START WITH THE FACILITY ITSELF

First impressions *do* matter, so pay attention. Your assessment should start with the facility's exterior. How and where is it situated? If it's on a busy street, check to see if it's set back from the road so it's safe and quiet. What is the building's condition as seen from the street? What do the grounds look like? Are they well kept? Are trees and bushes trimmed and lawns mowed? Is there litter around? Is the trash bagged neatly?

Take out a Medicare Nursing Home Checklist, the one found on the Internet or the one that follows here. It will help you focus on the details as you tour each facility.

THE NURSING HOME CHECKLIST

The Nursing Home Checklist

Use the Nursing Home Checklist when you visit a nursing home.
Take a copy of the Nursing Home Checklist when you visit to ask
questions about resident life, nursing home living spaces, staff,
residents' rooms, hallways, stairs, lounges, bathrooms, menus and
food, activities, safety, and care.

Use a new checklist for each nursing home you visit. You can
photocopy the checklist or print additional copies available at
www.medicare.gov/NHCompare.

Name of Nursing Home: _____

Address: _____

Phone Number: _____

Date of Visit: _____

Basic Information	Yes	No	Comment
Is the nursing home Medicare-certified?			
Is the nursing home Medicaid-certified?			
Does the nursing home have the level of care I need?			
Does the nursing home have a bed available?			
Does the nursing home offer specialized services, such as a special unit for care for a resident with dementia, ventilator care, or rehabilitation services?			
Is the nursing home located close enough for friends and family to visit?			

Visit Nursing Home Compare at www.medicare.gov/NHCompare for more information.

The Nursing Home Checklist

Resident Appearance	Yes	No	Comment
Are the residents clean, well groomed, and appropriately dressed for the season or time of day?			

Nursing Home Living Spaces	Yes	No	Comment
Is the nursing home free from overwhelming unpleasant odors?			
Does the nursing home appear clean and well kept?			
Is the temperature in the nursing home comfortable for residents?			
Does the nursing home have good lighting?			
Are the noise levels in the dining room and other common areas comfortable?			
Is smoking allowed? If so, is it restricted to certain areas of the nursing home?			
Are the furnishings sturdy, yet comfortable and attractive?			

Visit Nursing Home Compare at www.medicare.gov/NHCompare for more information.

The Nursing Home Checklist

Staff	Yes	No	Comment
Does the relationship between the staff and residents appear to be warm, polite, and respectful?			
Does the staff wear name tags?			
Does the staff knock on the door before entering a resident's room? Do they refer to residents by name?			
Does the nursing home offer a training and continuing education program for all staff?			
Does the nursing home check to make sure they don't hire staff members who have been found guilty of abuse, neglect or mistreatment of residents; or have a finding of abuse, neglect, or mistreatment of residents in the state nurse aid registry?			
Is there a licensed nursing staff 24 hours a day, including a Registered Nurse (RN) present at least 8 hours per day, 7 days a week?			
Will a team of nurses and Certified Nursing Assistants (CNAs) work with me to meet my needs?			
Do CNAs help plan the care of residents?			
Is there a person on staff that will be assigned to meet my social service needs?			
If I have a medical need, will the staff contact my doctor for me?			
Has there been a turnover in administration staff, such as the administrator or director of nurses, in the past year?			

Visit Nursing Home Compare at www.medicare.gov/NHCompare for more information.

The Nursing Home Checklist

Residents' Rooms	Yes	No	Comment
Can residents have personal belongings and furniture in their rooms?			
Does each resident have storage space (closet and drawers) in his or her room?			
Does each resident have a window in his or her bedroom?			
Do residents have access to a personal phone and television?			
Do residents have a choice of roommates?			
Are there policies and procedures to protect residents' possessions, including lockable cabinets and closets?			

Hallway, Stairs, Lounges, and Bathrooms	Yes	No	Comment
Are exits clearly marked?			
Are there quiet areas where residents can visit with friends and family?			
Does the nursing home have smoke detectors and sprinklers?			
Are all common areas, resident rooms, and doorways designed for wheelchair use?			
Are handrails and grab bars appropriately placed in the hallways and bathrooms?			

Visit Nursing Home Compare at www.medicare.gov/NHCompare for more information.

The Nursing Home Checklist

Menus and Food	Yes	No	Comment
Do residents have a choice of food items at each meal? (Ask if your favorite foods are served.)			
Can the nursing home provide for special dietary needs (like low-salt or no-sugar-added diets)?			
Are nutritious snacks available upon request?			
Does the staff help residents eat and drink at mealtimes if help is needed?			

Activities	Yes	No	Comment
Can residents, including those who are unable to leave their rooms, choose to take part in a variety of activities?			
Do residents have a role in planning or choosing activities that are available?			
Does the nursing home have outdoor areas for resident use? Is the staff available to help residents go outside?			
Does the nursing home have an active volunteer program?			

Visit Nursing Home Compare at www.medicare.gov/NHCompare for more information.

The Nursing Home Checklist

Safety and Care	Yes	No	Comment
Does the nursing home have an emergency evacuation plan and hold regular fire drills (bed-bound residents included)?			
Do residents get preventive care, like a yearly flu shot, to help keep them healthy? Does the facility assist in arranging hearing screenings or vision tests?			
Can residents still see their personal doctors? Does the facility help in arranging transportation for this purpose?			
Does the nursing home have an arrangement with a nearby hospital for emergencies?			
Are care plan meetings held with residents and family members at times that are convenient and flexible whenever possible?			
Has the nursing home corrected all deficiencies (failure to meet one or more state or Federal requirements) on its last state inspection report?			

Visit Nursing Home Compare at www.medicare.gov/NHCompare for more information.

The Nursing Home Checklist

Go to a resident council or family council meeting

While you're visiting the nursing home, ask a member of the resident council if you can attend a resident council or family council meeting. These councils are usually organized and managed by the residents or the residents' families to address concerns and improve the quality of care and life for the resident.

If you're able to go to a meeting, ask a council member the following questions and take notes:

- What improvements were made to the quality of life for residents in the last year? _____
- What are the plans for future improvements? _____
- How has the nursing home responded to recommendations for improvement? _____
- Who does the council report to? _____
- How does membership on the council work? _____
- Who sets the agendas for meetings? _____
- How are decisions made (for example, by voting, consensus, or one person makes them)? _____

Visit again

It's a good idea to visit the nursing home a second time. It's best to visit a nursing home on a different day of the week and at a different time of day than your initial visit. Staffing can be different at different times of the day and on weekends.

Notes on second visit: _____

_____

_____

_____

Visit Nursing Home Compare at www.medicare.gov/NHCompare for more information.

WHAT ELSE TO NOTICE

The Medicare Nursing Home Checklist does cover a great deal of information, but be sure to consider the following additional points too.

First, notice what residents are wearing. Long-term residents should be dressed in their own clothing. Patients who are sick, or who have been recently discharged from the hospital and are still getting IV fluids, for instance, might appropriately be wearing hospital gowns. That is acceptable; the gowns are easier for caregivers to work with. Just expect those gowns to be clean and dry.

Second, speak to residents and ask them how they like living at the facility. Your guide should certainly allow you to interact freely with them. If you see any visitors, strike up a conversation and ask what their experience with the facility has been. Don't forget to write down these observations in your notes.

Third, ask how resident roommates are assigned and what the procedure is for dealing with roommates who are incompatible.

Fourth, notice patient alarms, both audible alerts and lights. All residents should have a call button in their room that they can easily reach to press for help if need be. That button sounds an alarm and turns on a light at the nursing station. If you can, observe if those calls are being answered in a timely fashion. If you sense the calls are not being answered promptly, determine if there are competing issues that legitimately occupy the staff's attention. Keep observing this throughout your tour and on any follow-up visits.

Fifth, talk to staff members and pay attention to the nonverbal subtexts and cues in your conversations. Are they frank and open? Are staff members appropriately dressed and well groomed? Do they seem enthusiastic and interested in what they are doing? Ask how long have they been working at the facility. In particular, ask this question of nurses' aides and nurses, since they have the most day-to-day contact with residents. Unfortunately, turnover in these positions is normally high, so longevity would be surprising and a good sign. Also ask the aides how long they've been CNAs and how they feel about the facility itself and their work there.

MEALTIMES AND ACTIVITIES

Mealtimes—events occurring at least three times a day—provide opportunities to get residents out of their rooms. Ask your guide about the mealtime philosophy at the facility. For example, while patients have the right to refuse to take their meals with others, good nursing homes strongly encourage residents to leave their rooms to eat communally in the dining room. Why? Because going back and forth to the dining room is a form of physical activity, even if it's a matter of getting out of bed to be wheeled to the cafeteria in a wheelchair. Leaving the room also makes for a change of scenery, and is something residents can look forward to. After all, for most people, socializing is central to happiness. Mealtimes offer that opportunity.

After seeing where residents eat, find out where they go to smoke. There should be a designated area outside for smoking, if smoking is allowed at all. Even if your prospective resident is a non-smoker, you want to be assured that there will be no exposure to second-hand smoke.

Boredom and hopelessness set in if residents don't have a robust activities program to occupy them. Because activities are pivotal in a nursing home, meet the activities director and find out what's offered. Visit the activities room and learn what activities and outings are planned for the residents throughout the year.

What do they do in the facility? What individuals or groups do they bring in to entertain? Do they organize trips and outings away from the facility?

Nobody wants to be indoors all the time, so make sure each facility you visit has outdoor areas that you can see during your visit. Are staff members eager to assist residents out to those areas and chaperone them while there? Do they have more going on than bingo and a big-screen television? Regarding the activities program, you want to see that the facility has lots happening.

Many nursing homes have beauty shops on the premises. Often, the same people who work with women in the beauty shops also barber the men. You just want to know the details, how appointments are made, and what the costs are.

Be sure to inquire about the specifics of education and training the facility provides for its staff. *In-services* are training sessions conducted on-site for staff members. These can be sessions on procedures such as proper hand washing or the correct technique for lifting a patient into and out of bed.

Ask how often this kind of training session occurs. In a good facility, training is ongoing and frequent.

MEDICAL PROVIDERS

You will certainly want to know about the medical provider staffing arrangements—namely, the attending physicians and mid-levels (nurse practitioners and physician assistants) who make patient visits on-site.

Increasingly, more physicians' practices are collaborating with midlevel professionals to meet the growing demand created by the baby boomers; there just aren't enough doctors. We will be seeing more nurse practitioners and physicians' assistants in long-term care and other fields of medicine. Thankfully, their extra training and on-the-job experience qualifies them to handle most of the day-to-day issues nursing-home residents face.

First, be sure to learn how it works. There is a physician on hand and a medical director who oversees all medical-provider services at the facility.

Second, ask when medical providers make patient rounds. What is their accessibility after-hours and on weekends? It is unlikely your family member's current doctor will be able to make regular rounds at the facility, so take time to understand how the residents' medical-care needs will be met.

To be specific, check to see that the doctors, nurse practitioners, and physician assistants come into the building regularly, *not* sporadically. Do not expect their schedule to be identical to that required in a hospital where a doctor checks on each patient every day. Nursing-home medical providers check residents on a less frequent schedule. In the days soon after admission into a nursing facility, especially if a new resident comes in from a hospital stay, the medical provider will probably see that resident one to three times a week until the person stabilizes.

Naturally, the medical provider will not see each resident on every visit to the facility. Still, if something comes up, the medical provider will stop by and take a look.

STAFF WORK EXPERIENCE IS KEY

When making your nursing home tours, it's easy to be swayed by the appeal of new or renovated buildings and freshly redecorated interiors. A facility can have the fanciest equipment, but if staff members are always hurried and harried, or if they're not engaged in their jobs or not available when needed, no amount of equipment will make up for that. When you visit the rehab gym, don't only note what equipment is available; meet the therapists who work there. Staff work experience is the key. For your loved one's welfare, it's the staff members who will make or break patient-care outcomes.

To get to know them, ask how long they've been in their profession? How long have they been working in that facility? Do they seem to care about people? The best staff people are those who are more people-oriented rather than task-oriented. Good staff members know residents by name, not by medical condition, and will refer to Mr. Smith instead of "the pneumonia case in room 110." Chapter Six can guide you further.

STAY ORGANIZED

Be diligent in using a nursing-home checklist and make notes during your tour so you don't overlook the details or forget where you saw what. By recording your observations as you go, you can look back later and more easily make sense of that visit.

Also take photos to serve as memory joggers. Photograph a typical resident room, the dining hall, the activities room, the lounge, and so on. If your family member cannot make the site visit with you, sharing those photos helps you convey what you saw and keeps things straight for your own reference, too.

After the initial visits, you'll shorten your list to one or two places. You may or may not have the time or opportunity to make additional visits to those nursing homes on your family member's behalf. Sometimes events happen fast and it's necessary to move so quickly that taking a second look isn't feasible. In other cases, your schedule may make it impossible. That's all the more reason to take detailed notes, ask lots of questions, and view everything on your checklist the first time around.

Using these tools provides the assurance of knowing you have vetted the place as thoroughly as you could.

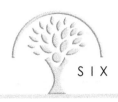

SIX

KNOW YOUR NURSING-HOME TEAM

Once you have found the right nursing home, and your family member has moved in, it's time to learn who's involved in giving the care.

Caregiving in nursing homes is a team approach. Teamwork, in nursing home care, is not just a slogan or platitude; it's true and put into practice daily. Facilities demonstrate the team approach in many different ways: executing as the **interdisciplinary team**, compiling the **minimum data set**, formulating **care plans** and presenting them, holding **stand-up meetings**, **signing out** at shift changes, and conducting **Quality Assurance** (QA) work and **meetings**.

Teamwork starts with an **Interdisciplinary Team** or the IDT. The IDT is a team of professionals who provide a comprehensive, coordinated assessment of each resident's medical, functional, and social needs in a nursing home. Federal regulations mandate using an IDT format in nursing homes. Each nursing home has to have a functioning one in place.

The IDT is made up of the facility's various department heads: the director of nursing, the head of the rehabilitation therapy department, the administrator, the director of social services, and the activities director. Within seven to fourteen days of any resident's admission to the nursing home, the team has to come up with a coordinated plan for the new patient.

The IDT works from an assessment form known as the **Minimum Data Set** (MDS). Each department has a section to complete on that MDS form in time for a team conference, called the care-plan meeting. Team members make time before the meeting to review the patient's medical record, interview the person and their family, and collect the required information. They each enter their data into the MDS and collectively come up with a care plan. For skilled-nursing/ short-term rehab patients, their data are collated within seven days of admission; for a long-term resident, their data should be all set by the fourteenth day. Federal law requires formulating these care plans, just as it requires IDTs.

CARE-PLAN MEETINGS

The team sets an initial care-plan meeting date and invites the patient, assuming he or she is not too cognitively impaired to participate meaningfully. A family member is also asked to attend or come in the resident's place. This keeps the family engaged in the patient's care, which is good for all involved. Meeting invitations are mailed and phoned in. As family members go in and out of the facility visiting the resident, staff will also tell them about the care-conference verbally.

Because this care-plan meeting is the official forum at which strategic decisions are made about treatment, it's important that someone from the family be there if possible. Unfortunately, care-plan meetings take place during regular working hours, which may make it difficult to attend if the responsible family member has a day job. Perhaps family members can rotate.

The first care-plan meeting should occur within thirty days of any patient being admitted into a nursing home. From that point on, it's conducted quarterly for as long as the patient resides there.

What is covered in this meeting? Essentially, the team presents the plan of care to the resident and their family. The plan addresses both medical and nonmedical issues, and outlines the goals of therapy, noting what outcomes are expected within what time frames.

It also lists which staff member is responsible for implementing and monitoring each aspect of the plan. For instance, a rehab goal might read, "Within thirty days, Mr. Sims will be able to walk 200 feet with a walker. The physical therapist on staff is responsible."

Of course, the patient and family members in attendance have the opportunity to ask any questions they may have.

MORNING MEETINGS

Another facet of the team approach is the daily **stand-up meeting** or **morning meeting** when all the heads of departments come together to confer. It's called a *stand-up* meeting because it's supposed to be so brief (lasting fifteen to thirty minutes), staff members don't even sit down!

At morning meetings, the administrator reviews what has happened overnight and previews what's coming up for the day ahead. Typical topics include transfers to the hospital, admissions the night before, deaths, accidents, and pending admissions. Have there been room changes? Did any grievances come up? By answering questions in this quick meeting, all the department heads receive updates on any changes or concerns.

TEAMS WORK IN SHIFTS

This team concept also plays out in the way staff members transition from shift to shift. There are three shifts: a morning shift, an afternoon shift, and a night shift. When staff members change shifts, they have to hand-off or **sign-out** patient-care duties. Those going off duty report to their counterparts coming on duty so details about patient care don't fall through the cracks.

QUALITY ASSURANCE MEETINGS

Teamwork is also demonstrated in **quality-assurance** (QA) work and **meetings**. QA is a federal requirement for nursing homes. The QA program deals with larger process and procedural issues that affect the operations of a nursing facility.

At QA meetings, high-level staff like the administrator, the director of nursing, and the other heads of departments come together monthly or quarterly, depending on the facility. A physician, the medical director, is part of the make-up of this committee. QA committees develop and implement appropriate plans of action to identify and correct quality deficiencies at a facility.

QA programs monitor trends in the following areas:
- pressure sores and skin breakdown
- psychoactive drug use
- transfers to hospitals

- medication errors
- bladder catheterization rates and catheter care
- weight loss and fluid intake
- infection rates
- depression
- restoration of function (e.g., following hip fractures)
- restraints
- falls resulting in injury
- abuse, neglect, and misappropriation of resident property

Taken together, all these team approaches are intended to provide the best possible care for residents.

INDIVIDUAL PROFESSIONALS ON THE TEAM

Who are the individual professionals in the nursing home and what do they do? How do you and your family member interact with them? The descriptions that follow explain.

Certified Nurses' Aides (CNAs): They are the unsung heroes in nursing-home care. Working under the supervision of nurses, CNAs provide hands-on personal-care assistance to patients who need help with some or all of their ADLs, which are bathing, feeding, dressing, transferring, toileting, and ambulating. They serve meals, record fluid and food consumption, provide skin care, and report changes in patients' conditions to nurses.

CNAs provide the first line of care and are key to patient satisfaction. To find out what's going on with a particular patient, go to their assigned nurses' aide. If you want an up-to-the-minute progress report on your family member, don't start at the top with the director of nursing. Instead, find the CNA and get the real scoop.

CNAs work hands-on with every patient. Even if a patient is capable of doing some things on their own, CNAs make sure those things get done properly. They have to document to what extent they assisted and record things like, "I stood by and watched Mr. Z put on his clothes, brush his teeth, and feed himself." "You can see that Mr. A is feeling better." "It took two of us to lift Mrs. B out of bed, put her in the shower-chair, and give her a shower."

Some CNAs take additional courses to become Certified Medication Aides (CMAs) and then focus on this line of work. "Med Aides" distribute medications, relieving LVNs to do more advanced nursing duties.

Licensed Practical Nurses (LPNs) or Licensed Vocational Nurses (LVNs): As the first level of nurses in the nursing home, these nurses take patients' vital signs, measure and track fluid input-output, and track food consumption. They also do wound care, handle feeding tubes, colostomies, and bladder catheters. They pass out medications, administer breathing treatments, and hang up IV fluids. Often, they're referred to as *charge nurses* because they are in charge of a wing or hall of the nursing home for a shift. In the nursing-home hierarchy, charge nurses are supervised by more experienced LVNs who hold Assistant Director of Nursing (ADON) positions.

Registered Nurses (RNs): In most nursing homes, registered nurses do not work on the halls the way LVNs do. Rather, because of their more extensive education, they're used administratively in MDS coordinator positions, other administrative roles, or ultimately as the director of nursing.

Director of nursing (DON): This person holds the top nursing position in a nursing home. An RN fills this role. The DON supervises all nurses and is the administrative head of nursing in the facility. As a big cog in the nursing-home wheel, the DON oversees the standards of nursing practices for the nursing home. He or she is in charge of developing protocols, programs, policies, and procedures to meet all state and federal requirements.

Social workers: These are professionals responsible to promote the residents' social and psychological well-being. They foster policies and an environment that enhances the patients' quality of life in respect to culture, religion, and ethnicity. In effect, they help those patients retain individuality and independence in the nursing home.

The social workers' job is also to make people comfortable and they take into account all the intangibles that clinical people may not focus in on. Typically, you first interact with a social worker during the admissions process. In addition to admissions, social workers are involved with discharges, and with making sure transitions happen smoothly without violating individual or cultural rights.

Social workers are on the lookout to see how a new resident is adjusting. If you are struggling with any guilt about putting your loved one in a nursing home, social workers are trained to spot that and can refer you to resources to help you work through your feelings. They're trained to spot and address a variety of considerations when putting a family member in a nursing home. You may well meet a social worker when you first tour the nursing home.

Social workers are often tasked with handling advance directives and will inquire if you have those documents in place. Advance directives are legal documents that allow you to convey your decisions about end-of-life care ahead of time. If no advance directives have been executed, social workers will pursue the matter and at least give you information on what is required to set up valid documents, even if you choose not to act on that information immediately. Whenever you do act, they'll work with you to see that the completed documents get to the right people for signatures.

A social worker attends each care-plan conference. Often, he or she screens residents for cognitive status, depression, and anxiety. And when a resident is discharged, a social worker arranges for home-health care and durable medical equipment.

Social workers serve as the liaison with home-health agencies and medical-equipment companies, getting people the services and equipment they need (nursing, physical therapy, wheelchairs, oxygen, and so forth).

Dieticians, nutritionists, or nutrition consultants: This professional plans the food and nutrition programs for the whole facility. In an oversight role, they are responsible for ensuring each patient is on the appropriate diet. A nutritionist goes into a nursing home on a regular basis to review patient weights and make appropriate recommendations.

The nutritionist's work also includes developing the prescriptions for complex feeding-tube diets; a specially trained professional must manage this complex prescription. Nutrition is a highly specialized field that requires years of education as well as continuing education to keep up with innovations.

Physical therapists, occupational therapists, and speech-language therapists: These professionals work for a nursing home's rehabilitation department with hands-on duties in the gym. The rehab department offers services to patients who have been discharged from an acute-care hospital stay. Patients are referred to rehab after planned surgery (e.g., a knee replacement), after emergency surgery (e.g., repair of a fractured hip, heart surgery for a heart attack, or appendix removal), or following an illness (e.g., a stroke, a bout of pneumonia, or an episode of congestive heart failure).

While the majority of rehab therapy patients tend to be short term, nursing staff can refer long-term patients for rehab if they detect a significant functional decline. Some nursing home rehab units also service patients living in the community—that is, they provide outpatient rehab. The goal of Rehab is to restore function and improve quality of life for patients, thus adding "life to years" in addition to adding "years to life."

The first members of the rehab team are the *physical therapists*—professionals who enhance patients' strength, range of motion, mobility skills, and endurance. Primarily concerned with promoting ambulation and transfers, they work their patients' big muscles on both upper and lower extremities. They may use electrical stimulation to enhance function or relieve pain.

Physical therapists teach patients to walk with canes or walkers or help them use a wheelchair. They also work with orthotics professionals who fashion braces for weak extremities and prosthetics experts who create artificial limbs.

Not primarily concerned with small-motor dexterity, physical therapists focus on the power and strength of their patients' upper and lower extremities. While occupational therapists are fine-motor-skill activity trainers, physical therapists help build patients' raw strength.

Occupational therapists (OTs) work on retraining patients with deficits in performing basic ADLs and IADLs. Specifically, they're concerned with fine-motor skills and dexterity: dressing, bathing, toileting, feeding, and so on. They also address cognitive issues. OTs can even help evaluate a patient's ability to drive a car.

While the term *speech therapist* suggests work with speech and communication, these professionals also play a major role in working with patients who have swallowing deficits and cognitive impairment. In terms of the speech process, these therapists mostly deal with nursing-home residents who have had strokes, late-stage dementia, and Parkinson's Disease.

As they grow older, many people find their swallowing is impaired in some way. Having a major illness exacerbates that problem. The main concern here is aspirating—that is, food going into the airways instead of the food pipe. This is a common problem among the elderly because the swallowing mechanism is made up of muscle, which becomes uncoordinated and weaker with age. Speech therapists are trained to teach patients certain exercises for the swallowing muscles that help overcome problems with swallowing.

Activity therapists are also unsung heroes in the nursing-home world where residents' challenges includes overcoming boredom. With each resident having different interests, the problem is compounded by the limited budget usually allocated to the activities department. A nursing home's activity director needs to be an organized, upbeat, enthusiastic, energetic person who has a creative mind. He or she has to devise art, music, dance, games, and craft programs that provide fun, education, and mental stimulation for the residents. The range of programming needs to be accessible for people with disabilities, illnesses, and cognitive problems. Having a strong activities program is key to keeping residents happy so they can avoid become introverted and disengaged.

The facility should have staff members rounding people up for activities. If they only announce the activities but leave it up to residents to get themselves out for it, residents may forget them or simply shrug off the opportunities.

When you tour nursing homes, pay special attention to the cultural values and to the activities department, especially when contemplating a long-term stay. In your moment of stress when placing your loved one in a nursing home, you likely won't be thinking about the activities available. Rather, you'll be focused on nursing and medical care. However, if your loved one lives in the home for a long time, the activities available will have a huge impact on the day-to-day quality of life. So when you visit facilities, take time to meet the activities director, look at the calendar of events offered, and find out about the culture itself.

Consultant pharmacists: Also called pharmacy consultants, pharmacists go into every nursing-home facility. While they may not be on site daily, every nursing home contracts with one to come in regularly and review medication regimens. These consultants pick up on potential drug interactions and communicate reminders about testing for medication blood levels. They recommend when it is time to taper down on doses or stop altogether. It is great teamwork to have these pharmacists cast a second set of eyes over the medications.

Nursing-home administrator: This person is the administrative head, the veritable CEO and head honcho of the facility. As the managing officer, the administrator is responsible for planning, organizing, directing, and controlling the facility's day-to-day functions and year-to-year progress. All department heads report to the nursing-home administrator who also runs the various meetings for the facility.

Attending physicians: These professionals have an important role to play. However, many aspects of care for nursing-home patients don't require direct physician input because they are not clinical in nature. This includes day-to-day personal-care assistance, nursing-care procedures, activities, socialization, and so on.

In the nursing-home setting, although physicians have a major role as part of the team, they aren't the center of this universe. Still, not too many things can happen without a physician's signature. For example, a patient can't be admitted into a nursing home without a physician's order nor can they be discharged without one. A physician also has to sign off on a dietary changes.

Staff members might change a patient's room because that's an administrative action, but most orders still actually receive a physician's signature. This could be considered rubber-stamping because some specialists (for example, nutritionists) know more about a particular area. Still, the law requires a physician to sign off on most orders affecting the health and well-being of patients. This authority is not necessarily superfluous because, of the all the professionals involved in the care of a patient, the physician is uniquely privy to all the moving parts (physical, mental, and social) and understands how they affect each other. Take a room change, for instance. You wouldn't want a recovered alcoholic moving in with a resident who is permitted a glass of wine every evening. Which professional is best positioned to connect the dots? The supervising physician.

Each resident in a nursing home is assigned a physician who looks out for medical necessity and regulatory policy. The policy is mandated by federal guidelines that specify each resident must be paid a certain number of visits, regardless of whether that individual has a medical complaint.

Specifically, a physician must visit a new patient on admission, then thirty days later, and then thirty days after that. Then visits become less frequent but shouldn't go longer than sixty days. Again, federal regulations dictate this schedule. Short-term patients who are more acutely ill than long-term ones usually need to be seen several times a week until they stabilize. The medical necessity rule applies here. (These are healthcare services that a physician exercising prudent clinical judgment would provide to a patient for the purpose of evaluating, diagnosing, or treating an illness, injury, disease, or its symptoms.

The medical necessity rule also allows for the medical provider's clinical judgment and discretion. This way, if something comes up between regulatory visits, the nursing-home patient is taken care of.

Nurse practitioners and physicians' assistants: Today, there are simply not enough physicians to adequately serve the nursing-home population, let alone the coming baby boomer surge. That's where *nurse practitioners and physicians' assistants* (midlevel providers) come in and make a tremendously valuable contribution. They have the clinical training to conduct patient visits, which are done in collaboration with a physician. Physicians are permitted to delegate certain regulatory visits and most medically necessary visits.

Medical director: Every nursing home is required to have a physician serving in a leadership and administrative role in the nursing-home organizational structure. The medical director position involves overseeing physician services as well as working with the administrator and director of nursing to ensure physician staffing and quality of care meet regulatory requirements. The best medical directors are certified as such by the American Medical Directors Association (AMDA).

AMDA—*the* professional association dedicated to long-term care—is a prestigious organization that issues a highly coveted certification, the Certified Medical Director (CMD) designation.

Other professionals: Facility Administrators can arrange for other professionals such psychiatrists, psychologists, podiatrists, optometrists, audiologists, and dentists to come in on consulting days. It's comforting to know your family member will have access to these specially trained people when they reside in a nursing home.

Psychiatrists and *psychologists* deal with mental health issues beyond the scope of the social worker and medical providers. A visiting *podiatrist* (a foot doctor) treats foot problems. An *optometrist* (an eye specialist) tests vision. An *audiologist* (a hearing specialist) tests hearing. A *dentist* comes in regularly to care for residents' teeth.

Hospice staff: Trained hospice workers are invited into a nursing-home facility to collaborate when a patient has a terminal illness and isn't expected to live beyond six months. In fact, many new patients may come into a facility already receiving hospice care.

A hospice team takes the lead in caring for a terminal patient. Sometimes existing residents decline gradually or take a sudden turn for the worse and require hospice care. Hospice workers have more experience, training, and resources than regular nursing-home staff to handle these special situations.

SPECIALIZED TEAM CARE

Let's again address the negative perception people have about nursing homes and the notion that hospitals "dump" difficult patients there. The descriptions of these professionals alone should lead you to reframe thoughts like these.

It's time to recognize that nursing homes are specialty institutions designed to help people who have complex medical issues. The specialized team care that's in place makes it all possible.

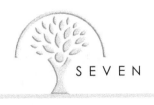

SEVEN

BE AN ADVOCATE FOR YOUR LOVED ONE

Your decision to move a family member into a nursing home may have been tough—perhaps even the most difficult decision of your life. In fact, you may feel you let your loved one down.

However, by accepting that you can't provide the care that person needs, you're putting your loved one's welfare ahead of your own ego. That, in itself, is advocating for your family member.

During his or her first week in the nursing home, you can do a lot to advocate for your loved one. The first few days can be particularly difficult and highly emotional as the new resident adjusts to the unfamiliar environment. Plan to be there as much as you can to lend support. Help unpack, hang up photographs, and decorate the room to make it feel cozy.

Nursing homes usually permit new residents to bring favorite things from home. That includes their own furniture when space allows. Certainly, your loved one can bring personal photos and small items. How much to include depends on whether the stay is short term or long term. If it's only for rehab, for example, bringing lots of personal items won't be necessary. However, if the stay is long term, bring as much as practical given the space provided.

CHECK OUT EATING OPTIONS TOGETHER

To acclimate your loved one to meals, check out the weekly menu together so he or she understands the choices available. Inquire not only about regular meals but about between-meal offerings. For example: "How does my husband get snacks?" "Are residents given drinks for hydration?" "How can my wife get ice or a cup of hot tea?" The CNAs can answer all of those questions. Nowadays, nursing homes often have food carts or snack stations that offer hot and cold drinks and snacks. Alternatively, the CNA brings these items to residents.

FIND OUT ABOUT ACTIVITIES—ESSENTIAL!

More than staving off boredom, a robust, varied selection of activities can stimulate, educate, and inspire people. Delve into what's available and make sure your loved one is aware of the possibilities. Find out where activities are posted (usually on a big board in the main lobby or in a hallway). Check to see if a calendar/flyer about activities and events is delivered to each room or posted on the wall or door. Take time to look over what's offered with your loved one and help identify activities of interest.

In addition, you might introduce yourself and your resident to the activities director and talk about outings or special events coming up. Remember, activities serve as more than time fillers; they offer enrichment that can make a bigger difference in a resident's life than all the clinical details.

LEARN ABOUT SERVICES ON-SITE

You might also take your family member to visit the on-site beauty shop or barber shop and meet the staff. Check out the amenities and services offered and ask how to make appointments. Together, you could establish a regular schedule for hair care on this visit. Find out if it's possible to get manicures, pedicures, and massage at the facility. They're a treat many people enjoy.

If your family member is religious, find out when and where worship services are held. Often, people take great comfort in their faith, and losing the connection with their regular place of worship can be a serious blow both spiritually and socially. See how you can facilitate new connections. You might take time to identify visiting clergy and arrange an introduction.

MEET NURSE'S AIDES

Get to know the certified nurses' aides (CNAs) who provide the most hands-on help a resident receives. They get residents out of bed, bathe them, and bring in meals if they can't go to the dining room. Ask which aide is assigned to your family member, then seek out that person and introduce yourself and your loved one. Ask about daily routines and other questions to help you get acquainted.

For some people who don't like to shower or have difficulty in the shower, bathing may be an issue. At times, the routine can seem quite regimented because the CNAs have to attend to everyone in a short amount of time. Some residents are so worried about getting cold that what should be a treat may not be enjoyable after all. Find out your loved one's preferences about bathing and how the facility might handle his or her requests. This will help allay any fears.

If your family member can't get in and out of bed without assistance, ask the CNAs how they typically do the required lifting. Depending on the situation, lifting may involve either one person assisting a resident (one-person assist) or two people (two-person assist). If the patient is particularly heavy, the task may require a mechanical lift device. As the advocate, you want to gather as much information as possible, both for yourself and your new resident.

ASK ABOUT MEDICAL ROUTINES AND EMERGENCIES

At what times do nurses pass out medications? How often do they check blood pressure and conduct a finger prick for blood sugar? What other procedures are available both routinely and with advance notice?

Confirm which physician has been assigned to your family member and find out when he or she comes in. Many doctors work with Nurse Practitioners and Physician Assistants as part of their nursing home practice team. Find out if this is true with yours and get to know them as well. Medical providers (physicians, nurse practitioners and physician assistants) may be in the building several days a week, but they won't see every patient each time. Learn how to get your family member attended to when the need arises. Also, understand that in nursing homes, by necessity, a lot of "telephone medicine" takes place. That is, the nurses call the providers and issues are handled over the phone. You want to be sure your loved one's assigned doctor responds promptly and regularly when called.

Every nursing home has contracts with laboratories for blood draws to be performed at the nursing home so residents don't have to go off-site. In addition, contracted mobile X-ray companies do simple X-rays on-site when the doctor orders them. Ask about these procedures and find out where residents go if they need a CT scan or some other high-tech test. What about transportation to these test appointments? Does a family or a staff member usually accompany residents on such an appointment? The answer to that question usually boils down to whether or not patients can comprehend and speak for themselves. For example, dementia patients may not be able to make their needs known. And stroke victims may have limited physical capabilities.

Ask the same questions for when appointments with a specialist (heart doctor, neurologist, kidney doctor, etc.) will be necessary. Make sure staff members at the nursing home have a contact list of the specialists your family member sees so they can set up appointments.

Also, find out how the nursing facility deals with emergency situations. Which hospital will your loved one be taken to, and how will he or she get there?

If your family member will be in the facility for rehab, visit the gym or exercise room and look into the routines. Together, examine the exercise equipment there. Ask questions. Who are the therapists? What days and times are therapy sessions? How long are the sessions? Get informed!

EASE THE SHIFT TO THE NEW FACILITY

If this seems like information overload to you, it will definitely feel overwhelming to your family member. However, if you proactively engage in this familiarization process, both of you will end up with a working knowledge of the new environment. This, in turn, is likely to greatly enhance your peace of mind and that of your loved one.

If you can't be with your new resident every day during the first week, take turns with other family members or friends if possible. Familiar faces make all the difference. If someone is present to support the transition, it will be less overwhelming and not such an alien experience for your family member. Nobody wants to feel written off. Your active engagement demonstrates your caring more than any words could ever do.

Don't be too discouraged if your family member initially shows distress or resists moving into this new environment. Different personalities have various degrees of difficulty adjusting to change. Over time, expect your family member to become familiar and comfortable with the new surroundings.

ATTEND CARE-PLAN MEETINGS

Another important way you'll be involved is to attend care-plan meetings. If your resident isn't too cognitively impaired, he or she will also be invited.

At the first care-plan meeting, the staff will present a comprehensive plan of care for your family member. You'll want to make sure everything staff members say is accurate and reflects a reasonable plan for your loved one. Your input matters. After all, you've known this person well for a long time, and the staff is just beginning to get acquainted with him or her. A staff member may say, "We'll take your mom down to the beauty shop once a month." If you know your mom likes her hair done every two weeks, speak up! Remember, this is a two-way discussion.

Perhaps the speech therapist has evaluated your loved one and recommends a ground-up diet. You know this option is intolerable to your family member. Be sure to discuss at the meeting the pros and cons of having a less restrictive diet to maintain quality of life, even if some risk is involved.

RESIDENT AND FAMILY COUNCIL MEETINGS

As an advocate, encourage your family member to attend the regularly held resident council meetings and you can go to family council meetings. At these meetings, the residents and families, respectively, get together with nursing home staff to discuss specific issues.

At resident council meetings, attendees focus on such topics as the facility's menu, housekeeping, social work, activities, and maintenance issues. These meetings are open for discussing anything concerning resident life.

As a member of the family council, you can influence, and be an advocate for, the well-being of your family member. It's a good idea to attend those meetings and encourage other families to attend too.

Remember, nursing-home residents who have a family member looking out for them in all respects have the best quality of life. Family members can help resolve everyday issues—from showers to laundry to hydration—when residents can't do so for themselves.

VISITS AND OUTINGS

Rather than having a set visiting schedule after that first week, pop in at different times. Attend an activity or drop in to chat. If it's physically possible for your resident to leave the nursing home, go on an outing; take your loved one to your home, a restaurant, or a family gathering. Remain active in their lives, and keep your family member involved in your life, too.

You'll feel better knowing you haven't "dumped" your loved one at a facility and you're actively looking out for him or her. That said, spread the responsibility around if you can, encouraging other family members to get involved so you don't burn out. If you can't visit your loved one because of a commitment, see if another family member or a friend can go. Part of your own involvement can be organizing a constant stream of visitors for your loved one.

At some point after that first week or two, it's okay to ease up on the daily visits. This will give your loved one time to become acclimated to the new situation and not use you as a crutch. Make sure your resident knows about the activities available while encouraging his or her participation.

KNOW YOUR LEGAL RESPONSIBILITIES

You'll also need to know about the legal aspects of being an advocate for your new resident.

Part of the nursing-home admissions procedure involves documenting the resident's responsible party (RP). Also the facility will want to note any advance directives the resident has in place, including a living will, medical power of attorney (POA), and Do Not Resuscitate (DNR) orders.

Responsible Party (RP): Many families think the "responsible party" is merely a contact person or the person with whom the nursing-home staff will discuss health care issues. However, this term in the nursing home's admission agreement pertains to *financial responsibility* for nursing-home bills. If you have the financial power of attorney for your family member, be sure to sign the agreement only as the "responsible party acting as the agent for…" Don't sign a legally binding contract that makes you financially liable for potentially huge expenses.

Advance Directives: These are various documents with written instructions regarding an individual's medical-care preferences. Family and medical professionals will consult these directives if that individual is unable to make his or her own health-care decisions. Advance directives include living wills, medical power of attorneys (POAs), and do not resuscitate (DNR) orders.

A *living will* is a legal document describing the types of medical treatment and life-sustaining measures an individual wants and doesn't want to receive. These procedures include intubation, mechanical ventilation, tube feeding, and resuscitation (such as CPR and electrical shock treatment).

A Medical POA is a legal document in which individuals designate family members or friends to make health-care decisions on their behalf in the event they're unable to do so for themselves. Medical information is confidential, so nursing-home staff want to know the right people (primary and secondary) in a family with whom to communicate information about the new resident. The chosen family member or friend is referred to as a *health-care agent, proxy, or Medical POA*. Medical POAs and financial POAs are separate documents with different purposes.

A *do not resuscitate order* (DNR) is another optional document. It's a request signed by the individual to not have cardiopulmonary resuscitation (CPR) if the person's heart or breathing stops.

Advance directives provide a cafeteria of choices; people don't need to have all three documents for any single one to be valid. Each document stands alone. However, a living will cannot cover every possible situation and decision. Therefore, a medical POA document designating a trusted person as a resident's health-care proxy is a good idea. From a clinician's standpoint, having all three documents provides the most solid framework for responsible actions.

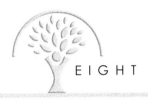

EIGHT

KNOW THE RIGHTS OF NURSING-HOME RESIDENTS

The day your family member enters a nursing home, you'll almost certainly receive a thick stack of paperwork. This includes everything from an activity calendar to an emergency-contact form and much more. In the stack will be a copy of the *nursing-home residents' bill of rights*. Like the U.S. Bill of Rights, it's not a document you and your resident are expected to consult daily. However, you do need to have some idea of what those rights are and where to lay hands on the document in the future. You may not have time to read the document at all that first day, but be sure to revisit it later.

To give you a jumpstart, this chapter explains the rights and clarifies them in the context of practice.

The rights of nursing home residents are usually codified in both federal and state statutes with the intent of further protecting each resident's civil, religious, and human rights while they reside in a nursing facility. The federal government guaranteed nursing-home residents' legal and moral rights in its 1987 reform law. The law requires nursing homes participating in the Medicare and Medicaid program to promote and protect the rights of each resident. It places a strong emphasis on individual dignity and self-determination. State laws for nursing home care usually mirror federal counterparts because the traditional standard of care for the nursing home industry is based on federal law. Some states have residents' rights written into *law*; others have *regulations* for nursing homes, assisted-living facilities, and other board-and-care facilities. If a nursing facility does not participate in Medicare or Medicaid, only state laws apply. Essentially, persons living in a long-term-care facility have the same rights as any individual living in the larger community.

Before reading the specifics about nursing-home residents' rights, you may want to take the following quiz just for fun to see how you do. (Answers are provided at the end of the quiz.)

FUN TRIVIA QUIZ: NURSING-HOME RESIDENTS' RIGHTS

1. Once individuals enter a nursing home, they lose their rights.
   a. True
   b. False

2. If a diabetic in a nursing home wants to have a piece of cake against the physician's orders, the nurse should…

   a. call the doctor for advice;
   b. give him or her something sugar-free;
   c. call the family for advice;
   d. allow him or her to have it.

3. Which of the following is NOT a right of a resident?

   a. getting drunk
   b. smoking
   c. masturbating
   d. carrying firearms

4. If a resident has food left on her face after a meal, is this a violation of her rights?

   a. yes

   b. no

5. If a man in a nursing home does not care for the food on the dinner menu, then...

   a. the kitchen should accommodate his choices;

   b. he will not be served dinner;

   c. his family will have to bring him something;

   d. he will have to eat it anyway.

6. If a woman does not want to take her blood pressure medicine, then...

   a. the nurse must get her to take it;

   b. she doesn't have to;

   c. she should be tied to her bed;

   d. the family must be informed.

7. If a nurse has put an elderly woman's hair in pigtails, and the patient did not ask for this hairstyle, does the situation violate her rights?

   a. no, because the woman couldn't do her own hair;

   b. no, because it looks attractive;

   c. yes, because it is not age appropriate;

   d. yes, because the nurse did it.

8. Technically, calling a resident "sweetie" or "honey" is a violation of someone's rights.

   a. true

   b. false

9. If a resident can no longer eat, a feeding tube should not be used if...

   a. a valid health-care proxy (chosen by the resident) gives such an instruction;

   b. a court-appointed guardian makes such a decision;

   c. if the resident stated such in a living will;

   d. any of the above.

10. If two residents are found to be openly engaging in intercourse, the facility should...

    a. turn a blind eye.

    b. consult a psychologist.

    c. ensure that neither party is being taken advantage of and require them to be more circumspect.

    d. put a halt to the whole situation by keeping them apart.

ANSWERS TO THE FUN TRIVIA QUIZ

1. b. False

2. d. Allow the person to have it. If a diabetic desires sugar, the staff should encourage diabetic alternatives, but if the patient continues to insist, it's his or her right to have the sugar.

3. d. Carry firearms

4. a. Yes. Leaving food on someone's face is a dignity issue.

5. a. The kitchen should accommodate his choices. Most nursing homes will accommodate any dietary request (vegetarian, kosher, etc.).

6. b. He or she does not have to. Residents have the right to refuse their medication.

7. c. Yes, because it is not age-appropriate. Again, this is a dignity issue.

8. a. True. Even though these pet names are well meant, they can be considered demeaning, so this is a dignity issue.

9. d. Any of the above

10. c. Ensure that neither party is being taken advantage of and require them to be more circumspect.

NURSING-HOME RESIDENTS' BILL OF RIGHTS

Under federal regulations, all nursing homes must comply with the following rights of residents.

1. **The Right to be Informed of Residents' Rights**

   The nursing home must have written policies concerning people's rights and responsibilities as residents. When admitted, a new resident must sign a statement saying he or she has received and understands these rights and the rules of the home.

2. **The Right to Be Informed about the Facility's Services and Charges**

   This includes charges for services not covered under Medicare or Medicaid and charges that aren't covered by the facility's basic rate.

3. The Right to Be Informed about One's Own Medical Condition

This is a right of every resident unless the physician notes in the patient's medical record that it's not in the patient's interest to be informed.

4. The Right to Participate in the Plan of Care

Every resident must be given the opportunity to participate in the planning of his or her medical treatment, including the right to refuse treatment.

5. The Right to Choose a Physician

Residents also have the right to choose their own pharmacy as well as physician. They don't have to use the nursing home's physician or pharmacy.

6. The Right to Manage Personal Finances

As a resident, an individual can either manage his or her own funds or authorize someone else to manage them. If a resident authorizes the home to handle his or her funds, the resident has the right to:

- know where the funds are and what the account number is.
- receive a written accounting statement every three months.
- receive a receipt for any funds spent.
- have access to the funds within seven banking days.

7. The Right to Privacy, Dignity, and Respect

Every resident has the right to be treated with consideration, respect, and full recognition of his or her dignity and individuality, including privacy in treatment and his or her personal care.

8. The Right to Use One's Own Clothing and Possessions

Residents may retain and use their personal clothing and possessions as space permits, unless to do so would infringe upon the rights of other patients or constitute a safety hazard.

9. The Right to Be Free from Abuse and Restraints

Every resident has the right to be free from mental and physical abuse and free from chemical and physical restraints except as authorized in writing by a physician. Then the restraints must be used for a specified and limited period or when necessary to protect the patient from injuring himself or herself or others.

10. The Right to Voice Grievances without Retaliation

Residents should be encouraged and assisted to exercise their right to voice grievances and recommend changes in policies and services to staff and/or outside representatives of their choice without fear of coercion, discrimination, or reprisal.

11. The Right to Be Discharged or Transferred Only for Medical Reasons or for One's Welfare or That of Other Residents

If either discharge or transfer becomes necessary, the resident must be provided with written notice 30 days in advance. Under law, residents have the right to appeal their discharge or transfer.

12. Your Rights of Access

- Residents may receive any visitor of their choosing and may refuse a visitor permission to enter their room or may end a visit at any time.
- Residents have the right to immediate access by family and reasonable access to others.
- Visiting hours of at least eight hours must be posted in a public place.
- Members of community organizations and legal services may enter any nursing home during visiting hours.
- Communication between the resident and visitor are confidential.
- Visitors may talk to all residents and offer them personal, social, and legal services.
- Visitors may help residents claim their rights and benefits through individual assistance, counseling, organizational activity, legal action, or other forms or representation.

The points in the sample Bill of Rights stated here are straightforward and self-explanatory. Some of the quiz answers may seem surprising, but if you give them open-minded thought, you will likely find they make sense in the spirit of self-determination.

FREEDOM FROM ABUSE, NEGLECT, AND EXPLOITATION

Treating residents with dignity follows from the principle that facilities should be free of abuse, neglect, and exploitation. This means that nursing-home staff should not shout at or otherwise harass residents; they must treat residents with respect. For example, some people like to be addressed by their first name; others more formally. All staff caring for residents should call them by their preferred names.

The hygiene of a resident's surroundings is both a dignity issue and a health issue. Staff must clean a resident's room on a regular basis and make the bed every day. If a resident soils the bedding, it must be changed as soon as possible. If a resident uses a bedpan, it should not languish there, dirty, in the room. It must be emptied and replaced in short order. The home's public spaces and exterior also fall under this rule; they, too, need to be clean and in good order.

Avoiding *neglect* comes down to common sense. If a resident is placed on a bedpan, for example, he or she should not be left there for an hour. Staff must go back after a short interval to check on the patient.

The same consideration applies to shower times. The air can be cold at times, even in warm regions of the country. Shower rooms in particular tend to be drafty. Aides on shower duty should ensure residents are wrapped up and warm while waiting for their turn to shower. If the process isn't accomplished smoothly and quickly and a resident complains of being cold on repeated occasions, that could be construed as neglect.

Another shower issue is water temperature. The water needs to be the right temperature for each resident; if it's not, that could be considered abuse. Shower aides should strive to accommodate a patient's preference.

Exploitation relating to nursing homes refers to the fact that the residents' personal belongings should be safe from theft and pilfering—even from family. The facility administrators should step in to handle the situation.

Family members could be misappropriating the resident's social security checks and other funds. There are situations in which residents have been brought to a nursing home by Adult Protective Services. In such cases, facility staffers need to know who was exploiting these patients on the outside so they can protect their charges.

Residents must be free from *discrimination* based on age, race, religion, sex, nationality, disability, marital status, and source of payment. Today, people with all sorts of religions, nationalities, and cultural differences live in nursing homes. Therefore, facility employees are required to be aware of and respect these differences.

A relatively common issue that may come up relates to Jehovah's Witnesses who don't want to receive blood products, or with Muslims who pray several times a day. This kind of information should be in the residents' chart so nursing-home staff members are aware of it and can respect the residents' rights. This awareness applies to religion-based food preferences, too.

Residents should be permitted to practice their own religious beliefs. Staff members need to know and respect that people differ in their beliefs and do things differently. Even visiting physicians are not exempt. They may plan to go into a resident's room on rounds, but if that resident is engaging in a religious rite, the physician should not interrupt but simply come back later.

This religious freedom also means residents can arrange for their own clergy to come in and perform rites as long as the practice doesn't infringe on other residents' rights.

The ninth rule on our list of residents' rights—to be free from abuse and restraints—is a big one. This right covers a broad spectrum of both physical and chemical restraints. Even the decision to use bedrails must be carefully weighed by the facility's staff on a case-by-case basis; bedrails could be considered restraints.

While hospitals have different and less stringent rules, in a nursing home, the issue of restraints is both tricky and sticky. Even a cushion that makes it more difficult for a resident to get out of a wheelchair could be considered a restraint. Staff members need to think of residents' safety first; the potential restraint can't primarily be for their convenience.

The same applies to medications or chemical restraints. If a resident is agitated a lot, the question to consider is, "Should we give this resident something to calm down?" To make that call and abide by the law, staff members have to evaluate if the resident is in danger of harming himself/herself or others without the medication. If not, there's a fine line between calming the patient down and mitigating inconvenience for the staff.

This rule requires staff members to try all the non-medicinal solutions they can to ameliorate the problem before choosing the medication option.

FREEDOM OF CHOICE

Several of the rules fall into the realm of a resident's freedom of choice.

If they have the mental capacity to do so, residents have the right to make their own choices regarding personal affairs, finances, and services. They have the right to choose their own physician, too. When patients move into a nursing home, they often want to know if their current community doctor can continue to be their doctor in the nursing home. The answer depends on whether their doctor will come to the nursing home regularly and be responsive to staff phone calls. However, it's rare that doctors who have busy clinic practices are willing or able to leave their offices regularly to see a nursing-home resident. If the physician can't or won't continue as the patient's primary-care physician, the resident must choose someone else from the nursing home's roster.

New residents are presented with a list of doctors who make rounds at the facility. While they won't know those doctors, the staff can serve as surrogate references. Residents or their medical power of attorney (POA) can choose. The key is that residents are presented with choices.

FREEDOM TO COMPLAIN

Another important residents' right is the ability to complain and be heard, as outlined in number 10 on our list.

This right also guarantees that residents will be safe from any reprisals if they do bring up a problem. A common example is complaints about the quality of the food or the level of assistance received with feeding. Another common problem concerns residents not getting along with their assigned roommate. Complaints often also come from family members. For example, they might think their loved one is not receiving enough therapy or some other service.

During your scouting facility tour, you may have interpreted staff members comments about what they'd do for your family member a certain way, and you may have chosen the nursing home based on that understanding. Later on, however, you may think those services aren't being rendered. These kinds of issues arise every day; they have to be arbitrated.

RESOLVING DISAGREEMENTS

How do you resolve the inevitable disagreements and disputes that come up between residents and nursing facilities? Rather than knowing the minute details about each section of the residents' bill of rights, it's much more useful to know what steps you can take to resolve issues.

It's best to work your way up the hierarchy of authority. If the problem relates to personal care or nursing, first speak to the CNA (for personal care), then the charge nurse, then the ADON, and finally the DON. If the problem is medical, speak with the charge nurse who can get a message to the physician's team. Lastly, if the problem involves administration, talk to the nursing-home administrator.

If you don't achieve resolution in this informal manner, bring the topic up at one of the regularly scheduled care-plan meetings. Each department will be represented at that gathering. Of course, if the issue is too urgent to wait, you can request a special family meeting. Keep in mind that for almost any situation, you can always run things by the facility social worker who will advocate for your family member.

So far, all of these attempts to resolve the situation take place at the nursing-home level. If you've exhausted all these channels and your issue is still not resolved, you can contact your local or state long-term-care ombudsman and air your complaints or request. As your advocate, the ombudsman and will act on your resident's behalf. Ombudsmen are assigned to several nursing homes in a locality.

To find contact information for the ombudsman program in your state, go to www.ltcombudsman.org/ombudsman.

If the issue constitutes a violation of residents' rights and the hierarchy of simpler measures doesn't resolve it, you may have to make a formal complaint to the nursing home licensing agency in your state. Be aware that doing so will trigger an on-site investigation. Calling for such action constitutes a serious step, thus one that's not to be taken lightly. The state investigators may not limit their investigation to your resident's complaints; at their discretion, they could expand the inquiry.

Beyond governmental resources but short of legal counsel, you could hire a geriatric-care manager to mediate the situation. This would bring in an advocate who's not personally involved and who understands how nursing homes function. Serving as an intermediary with the nursing home, the geriatric-care manager can help you determine what's possible.

Your second-to-last option, which is very rare, is to hire an attorney if the situation appears to be irresolvable without legal action. While an attorney may be necessary to assert a resident's rights, that attorney's involvement may also escalate the dispute to the point of being more difficult to resolve out of court.

Ultimately, you may determine that the facility cannot or will not meet your resident's needs. Because your main concern is getting your family member's issue resolved, it may be best to move your loved one to another facility. Doing so doesn't mean you can't still pursue legal recourse through an attorney, but you do want to have peace of mind. You don't want to stay worried about your family member's welfare and comfort because of an ongoing dispute.

Every nursing home should have a copy of the residents' rights posted for all to view. Your loved one's rights include being informed about these rights! If the facility doesn't have a copy of the rights on the wall somewhere, ask for a copy. And don't be afraid to speak up if you feel your loved one's rights are not being respected.

It should be recognized that, in an institutional setting, each and every resident cannot have complete freedom. However, facilities should go to great lengths to respect individual choices. These include sleeping patterns, food likes and dislikes, flexibility in bathing times, religious preference, clothing choices, friendships, and more.

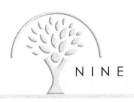

NINE

PAYING FOR NURSING-HOME CARE

Nursing home care is not only an emotional hurdle, it's a financial one as well. Half the battle is figuring out how all the expenses will be handled because you'll probably have to use more than one funding source to cover the full cost.

Typically, no single health-insurance option is going to pay for all of the nursing home costs. Each insurance plan has its own rules and coverage, which can be confusing. The ambitious intent of this chapter is to attempt to simplify it all and provide you with some tools (illustration tables) you can revisit over and over again.

Note: Because the fine details of health insurance for nursing-home care is unavoidably complex, it's probably not worth worrying about them. Take comfort in knowing that the experienced staff—both at the hospital and the nursing facility—can help you figure out all you need to know about your loved one's specific medical insurance benefits related to nursing-home care.

If you do want to dive in yourself, first be aware that payment for a nursing-home stay depends on whether it's a *short-term stay* or a *long-term stay* because the sources of payment are different.

Recall that a short stay, when a patient needs skilled nursing care and/or rehabilitation therapy, lasts from days to weeks. The other short-stay situation is when a patient is expected to live no longer than six months and is enrolled in hospice care.

Long-term placement is indicated for a person whose functional status in the community is handicapped. It's also for those who don't have adequate family support or the financial means to hire caregivers to take care of their ADL and IADL needs at home.

A second factor to consider is the breakdown of what needs to be paid for into different categories. The three categories include: *nursing-facility room and board, physician services, and medication costs.* Each one may be covered wholly, partially, or not at all, depending on the insurance policy.

It may help you to see all this information in one place, so begin by examining the two tables that follow. The first table summarizes payment options for a short-term stay; the second does the same for a long-term stay.

Paying For Nursing Home Care
Skilled Nursing Rehab Therapy (Short Stay)

Source of Payment	Room & Board	Physician Services	Medication Costs
Medicare/ "Traditional Medicare" (MCR)	MCR A	MCR B	MCR A
Medicare Managed Care/ Medicare Advantage Plans	*"Each company's policies vary"*	*"Each company's policies vary"*	*"Each company's policies vary"*
Private/ Commercial Health Insurance	*"Each company's policices vary greatly, differing in eligibility, restrictions, costs & benefits"*	*"Each company's policies vary"*	*"Each company's policies vary"*
Medi-Gap/ Medicare-Supplement	*"Depending on the plan, partially or fully covers coinsurance"*	*"Depending on the plan, partially or fully covers copays, coinsurance, deductible, & excess charges"*	*"Not applicable"*
Veterans (VA) Benefit	*Covers at VA medical centers & nursing homes with VA contracts*	*Limited coverage if not a VA doctor*	*Covers if obtained from VA sources*

Paying For Nursing Home Care
Non-Skilled Care i.e., Custodial Care (Long Term)

Source of Payment	Room & Board	Physician Services	Medication Costs
Medicaid/ "Nursing Home Medicad" (MCD)	MCD	MCD	MCD
Medicare (MCR)	*"No Coverage"*	*"Not applicable"*	*"Not applicable"*
Long-Term Care (LTC) Insurance	LTC Ins	*"Not applicable"*	*"Not applicable"*
Private Payment (PP)/ Personal Funds/ Out-of-Pocket	PP	*"Not applicable"*	*"Not applicable"*
Veterans (VA) Long-Term Care Benefits	VA LTC *(covers if VA facility or nursing home with VA contract)*	VA LTC *(limited coverage if not a VA doctor)*	VA LTC *(covers if obtained from VA sources)*
Medicare Managed Care (MCR C or MCR Advantage Plans)	*"Each company's policies vary"*	*"Each company's policies vary"*	*"Each company's policies vary"*

In the table for short stays under the column labeled "Source of Payment," the list includes the following: Traditional Medicare, Medicare Managed Care (Medicare Advantage Plans), Private/Commercial health insurance, Veterans' Benefits, and Medigap insurance.

In the second table, the payors for long-term stays are the following: Nursing Home Medicaid, Medicare (which has a limited role in long stays), Long-Term Care insurance policies, Private Payment (out-of-pocket, personal funds), Veterans' Long-Term Care benefits, and Medicare Managed Care. Note that the two lists of payor sources are quite different.

Seniors 65 years of age and older probably have traditional Medicare or a Medicare managed-care plan. Individuals younger than 65 may have private insurance or no insurance at all. In the case of younger patients without any insurance at all, they could still receive skilled nursing care and/or rehabilitation therapy either in a safety-net hospital system or in a nursing home that has a contract with a hospital and receives charitable funds from them.

WHAT IS MEDICARE AND WHAT DOES IT COVER?

Medicare provides health insurance for seniors 65 years of age or older, people under 65 with certain disabilities, and individuals of any age with End-Stage Kidney Disease. Medicare has four parts, each covering different, specific services: Medicare Part A, Medicare Part B, Medicare Part C, and Medicare Part D.

Part A covers inpatient care in hospitals, skilled nursing-facility care *(including room and board, medications, but not physician services)*, hospice services, and home-health care.

Part B covers physician services *(including nursing home visits)* and other health-care-provider services, hospital outpatient care, durable medical equipment (wheelchairs, scooters, lift chairs, walkers, etc.) and home health care. Part B also covers many preventive services.

Part C is Medicare Advantage or Medicare managed care. These are health-plan options run by private insurance companies that have permission from Medicare to compete with traditional Medicare. One well-known example of a Medicare managed-care plan is Secure Horizons. In addition, all the major commercial insurers such as Aetna, Humana, and Anthem Blue Cross/Blue Shield have Medicare advantage plans. Medicare managed-care does cover both short stays and long stays in nursing homes, but *policies vary from company to company*. Note: These plans offer wide and differing scopes of services too complex to address here.

Part D covers prescription medications. Medicare-approved private insurance companies run these plans. *Part D coverage is not needed by patients during a short-term nursing-home stay because Part A will cover medications in that situation. However, Part D does come into play in the long-term cases.*

SHORT-TERM STAY COVERAGE

To qualify for Medicare to pay for a short-term stay (skilled-nursing and/or rehab therapy), the potential resident must have Medicare insurance and must have spent three or more days in an acute-care hospital. Technically, this involves a minimum of "three inpatient midnights." While that patient was in the hospital, he or she must have received skilled medical services, not just testing (e.g., an MRI, cardiac stress testing) or other minor procedure (e.g., getting a G-tube put in or having a hemodialysis fistula created). A physician has to certify that the patient needs to continue skilled-nursing care in a nursing home, or that the person needs rehabilitation therapy after the hospitalization.

To qualify, the patient's admission to the nursing home has to be within 30 days of the hospital stay.

Even when health care professionals recommend skilled nursing and rehabilitation, some patients insist on going home after they've been in the hospital. Then, after they've been at home for a while, they realize they can't manage on their own after all. However, with the appropriate physician's order, they can still get into a nursing home for skilled nursing and rehab *if they're admitted within 30 days of the hospital stay.*

Let's say a senior qualifies for a skilled-nursing-home short-term stay and is admitted. If that senior has Medicare Part A, days 1 through 20 will be covered 100 percent for room and board costs, medications, and tests the doctor orders. No copayment is required from the patient during this duration (days 1 to 20). From day 21 through day 100, Medicare Part A will cover 80 percent of the bill. For the remaining 20 percent of the bill, the patient needs either a Medigap policy or personal funds. For all 100 days, the patient also needs to have Part B to cover the cost of physician services.

Instead of traditional Medicare, a senior might have chosen a Medicare managed-care plan for health insurance. Such a plan could pay for a resident's nursing-home stay including room and board, medications, and physician services. Remember, though, that specific coverages of the various companies policies differ significantly.

Military veterans can use their veterans' health benefits to cover a short-term stay for skilled nursing and/or rehab. That stay usually has to be in a veterans' facility, but some nursing homes have contracts with the VA system to provide skilled nursing and rehab to veterans.

What about someone younger than 65? To receive nursing home coverage, that person would need to have private/commercial insurance that specifically covers short-term nursing-home stays. Most private insurance plans have limited (sometimes greatly limited) nursing-home coverage. They definitely don't cover as much as Medicare does, and plans vary greatly in eligibility requirements, restrictions, costs, and benefits.

LONG-TERM STAY COVERAGE

Payor sources for the long-term coverage include: Nursing Home Medicaid, Medicare in a limited fashion, long-term care insurance, private payment (out-of-pocket, personal funds), veterans' long-term benefits, and some managed Medicare plans.

To be clear, Medicare does not serve as a major payor in the permanent placement arena. Medicaid is the big payer of residential nursing-home care.

If a patient who has limited income or very little means stays in a nursing home for the long term, Medicaid is the primary insurance. In that scenario, it covers room and board, physician services, and medications. Medicaid, which is state-funded insurance, pays for 7 out of 10 people who are long-term care residents in nursing homes, and highly complex rules determine who qualifies. If you have few financial means, your low-income status qualifies you. If you have some resources and some positive net worth, regulations require you to "spend down" your assets before you can qualify for Medicaid. The rules regarding spending down are complex and beyond the scope of this book.

If the patient has personal means or a long-term care insurance plan, room and board can be covered that way; Medicare B or Medicare C can be purchased to cover physician services; Medicare D or Medicare C will cover medication costs.

Individuals who have significant personal wealth can afford to pay out of pocket for room and board. To pay for physician services and medications, they usually have health insurance.

Long-term care insurance covers room and board in a nursing home for a long-term stay but usually not for a short-term stay. However, the patient still needs to have either Medicare or private insurance to cover physician services and medication costs.

In the past, not too many people purchased long-term care insurance policies, but nowadays these plans are becoming increasingly popular.

Referring again to the Paying for Nursing-Home Care table (long stay), the final option is Medicare managed care. Managed Medicare is an alternative to Medicaid in long-term cases, depending on the details of each policy.

Veterans' benefits have become more standardized. A long-term care package is available for military veterans who go into nursing homes permanently. This applies to VA facilities or nursing homes that have a contract with the VA as more veterans need permanent placement than the VA facilities can support.

PLAN AHEAD FIVE YEARS AT LEAST

Nursing-home expenses mount up fast. The cost of a nursing-home stay is somewhere between $60,000 to $75,000 a year, for room and board alone.

If you have the means, you need to consult an attorney who specializes in this area of eldercare to guide you through the process. It's prudent to plan a minimum of five years ahead of any possible need so you can protect your assets as much as possible.

Most nursing homes accept Medicaid, but some don't. If you need it and qualify for it, be sure to check before you choose a home. By and large, those homes that don't accept Medicaid are facilities looking for patients who can pay for rooms privately or use long-term care insurance. Some facilities have the complete mix (short-stay, long-stay, private pay, and long-term care insurance). When you're touring nursing homes, find out this information. Otherwise, if you put your family member in one for a short-term stay, you may have to move your loved one to another facility if the stay becomes long term.

Even though paying for nursing-home care is complicated, you most certainly will not be on your own when putting it all together. Certain staff members in the nursing home (e.g., the social worker, administrator, and director of nursing) will help you figure it out. In addition, the administrative personnel who deal with billing understand the details. In fact, it's part of the admissions process to determine what resources you or your family member may have: Medicare, Medicare managed care, Medigap policies, and so forth.

This chapter isn't intended to provide an exhaustive treatise on paying for nursing-home care. Rather, it provides the framework to understand nursing-home finance as it applies to patients. Conducting advance planning with an attorney or a financial planner can solve many potential financial issues before they occur.

If possible, don't wait for an emergency to make your contingency plan. Then if and when a nursing home becomes necessary, let knowledgeable hospital and nursing-home staff go over your health insurance benefits with you. It's like the relationship between electricity and a light switch; you don't have to understand how it all works to make the best use of it.

The baby boomer juggernaut is here. You may have already been affected by it, pulled in because of a spouse, parent, grandparent, uncle, or aunt needing nursing-home placement. If not, you may well be in the near future. The sheer volume of this demographic will put a strain on the health-care system, including hospitals, doctors' offices, and long-term care (LTC) facilities like nursing homes.

This book has addressed the LTC field. It explained the long-term care continuum, including:

- senior centers,
- adult day cares,
- home-health services,
- hospice services,
- assisted-living/memory-care centers, and
- nursing homes—both skilled-nursing facilities (SNFs) and nursing facilities (NFs).

Despite the move to develop and grow community-based services, our focus has been on SNFs/NFs. These nursing-home services are least understood, most misunderstood, and not going away anytime soon.

Nursing homes care for America's most chronically impaired and disabled individuals, subacutely ill patients discharged from hospitals, and recovering surgical patients. The topic is valuable to clarify because of:

- the inevitable growth of the age group that most needs nursing-home care
- the public's unfamiliarity with these matters
- the government's reluctance to deal with Medicare-Medicaid and its ignorance about long-term care and the nursing-home world.

Ultimately, this book succeeds if it makes LTC a household word and increases awareness about nursing home care *before* services are needed. An *informed* consumer is an *empowered* consumer.

The book has discussed the two major groups in nursing homes: short-stay patients and long-term residents. *Short-stay residents* are recent hospital patients recovering from medical illnesses or surgery who need skilled nursing care and/or rehab therapy.

Long-term residents either make the transition to permanency after an intended short stay, or they're admitted initially with long-term intent. Both groups have limitations on their activities of daily living (ADLs) that family and community resources can't meet. The limitations of those in a short-stay facility are expected to be temporary, whereas the limitations of residents in long-stay situations are permanent. Most long-stay individuals end up in nursing homes when two or more ADLs can't be managed at home or in the community.

Entry into a nursing home is often rushed rather than deliberate and controlled, but it needn't be. In the hospital setting, case workers, discharge planners, and social workers are wonderful resources in the search for nursing homes. In the community, a doctor's office staff, family, friends, and social-group referrals can serve as starting points. Out in the community, professional geriatric-care managers coordinate placements.

If you feel comfortable searching online, Medicare's Nursing Home Compare website is a useful and informative resource to investigate. It offers a downloadable checklist you can use in your onsite nursing-home tours (a must). A checklist can help you stay organized at individual facilities and compare different facilities. Remember the most important priorities: neat, clean surroundings and friendly, knowledgeable staff, not necessarily brand-new buildings, décor, or equipment.

Once you've selected a nursing home and gained admission for your loved one, doubt and guilt may bubble up. However, if you've exhausted family and community resources and consulted your health team to this point, you've probably made the right decision and best choice.

Stay strong; your loved one still needs you at this time. Coordinate the move-in; get to know the staff and routines; learn how to make things happen on a day-to-day basis; and learn the grievance process.

A nursing home placement may not be ideal, but it may be the right thing to do to care for yourself or your loved one.

FORTY-SEVEN TIPS FOR GUARANTEEING YOUR LOVED ONE THE BEST POSSIBLE OUTCOME

The following 47 tips provide guidelines in a nutshell to help you:
- find the right placement for your family member,
- understand what goes on in a nursing home,
- be aware of the rights of nursing home residents,
- make the transition as easy on everyone as possible.

GENERAL POINTS

1. **Consider the patient's priorities when determining that nursing-home care is necessary.** The amount of nursing care and supervision dictates the kind of facility best suited for the patient. Most nursing homes have sections for both short-term and long-term stays.

2. **Expect skilled-nursing beds to be the solution for short-term care.** These beds are usually for patients who are coming out of acute hospital care who still need skilled nursing care. These patients may also be permanent nursing-home residents who got sick, were transferred to a hospital, and are returning to a skilled-nursing bed in the facility.

3. **Understand that the goal is for skilled-nursing patients to be discharged to their homes again after illnesses such as:**
   - severe pneumonia
   - severe urinary tract infection
   - heart attack
   - stroke
   - hip, knee, or shoulder replacement
   - heart surgery
   - gall bladder removal

4. **Realize that a patient is a candidate for a long-term nursing-home stay when he or she needs help with two or more ADLs.** These activities of daily living include:
   - bathing
   - dressing
   - eating
   - grooming
   - transferring
   - toileting

5. **Recognize that a nursing home is ideal for people who cannot find care elsewhere.** This larger definition of care includes shelter, food, basic care, and a secure environment.

6. **Look to a nursing home as a good solution for the elderly or people of any age who have been previously isolated.** This can open up exciting opportunities in terms of social contacts and activities.

7. **Accept that nursing homes are set up to manage confused, violent, and mentally impaired patients.** The facility provides therapy and offers protection to the community at large.

8. **Find relief in relocation to a nursing home when your family has struggled with a heavy burden of physical caregiving.** This can free your energy to meet your loved one's emotional needs.

CHOOSING THE BEST PLACE

9. **Talk to those you know for their input.** Whether they know the patient or not, they know you, and they have a feel for your medical and general living needs. These people include your doctor, social worker, hospital discharge planner, family, friends, or others who could be helpful. They can often be objective and may have useful personal experiences to share.

10. **Work from a thorough checklist.** See the "Consumer Resources" section of this book for guidance on accessing an excellent, in-depth checklist.

11. **Choose a nursing home that's close enough for family and friends to visit.** It's important for your loved one to have visitors and also important for you to make the situation as workable for your own life as possible. You can search for nursing homes by city, county, state, or ZIP code as well as name. See the Medicare link in the "Consumer Resources" section of this book.

12. **Understand that nursing-home ownership is divided into for-profit, not-for-profit (e.g. Masons, Good Samaritans, religious orders, professional unions), or government-owned (e.g., VA) organizations.** Nursing-home ownership may be important in your search, especially if a personal affiliation offers an advantage to the potential resident.

13. **Consider any special services required that the nursing home would need to provide.** These services could include the following:

    - dementia care
    - ventilator units
    - bariatric care
    - rehab units
    - other specific services

14. **Make sure the nursing home has the level of care needed.** This can include skilled-nursing-facility beds, Medicare-certified beds, Medicaid-certified beds, and custodial (long-term) beds.

15. **Visit the nursing home more than once.** You will get a more realistic perspective by visiting at different times of day and with short notice. Have someone else visit for you if you're unable to do so yourself.

BEFORE MAKING A FINAL DECISION

16. **Contact the long-term ombudsman or state survey agency in your state.** Although your research may have been very

thorough, these people can sometimes shed light on something you hadn't considered.

17. **Realize that the more individualized and less regimented the required care for your loved one, the less the facility will look like an institution and the more it will look like a home.** That includes differences in layout and appearance. Some places have plants and resident animals, and sometimes children visit. These elements have been shown to bring greater happiness to the residents and their families.

18. **Understand that, generally, the more homey the look and feel of a nursing home, the higher the price will be.**

19. **Determine if the care is more task-oriented or resident-oriented. Resident-centered staff members know residents by name.** Institutionalized, task-oriented staff members identify residents by room number, diagnosis, or tasks for residents who need help. As you would imagine, resident-oriented care provides patients with a higher quality of life, although it has not been shown to lengthen the patient's life.

WHAT MATTERS MOST

20. **Look at the residents' appearance to be sure they're clean, well groomed, and appropriately dressed.** Dignity is a crucial part of overall well-being and needs to be respected, encouraged, and supported. In fact, it's a right of every nursing home resident.

21. **Notice the general environment.** A place that's well-lit and tidy, with a reasonable noise level, is inviting for everyday living.

22. **Observe how happy the people are and how homey the place feels.** After all, the place you choose will be your loved one's home—perhaps for a long time.

23. **Think about whether your loved one would rather live in a large nursing home with several hundred residents or a smaller facility with fewer services and activities but more personal attention.** Also consider whether a private room is a requirement or sharing a room is acceptable. Individual preference matters.

24. **Use the tool at the Medicare site listed in the "Consumer Resources" section of this book to compare the quality of the nursing homes you're considering.** You'll find information there on overall ratings, health inspection results, nursing-home staff data, quality measures, and fire-safety inspection results.

25. **Find out whether smoking is allowed.** If so, is it restricted to a particular area? Is that situation satisfactory to the future resident?

26. **Talk with the staff members.** You'll quickly discern if they're warm, polite, and respectful to the residents. While their training and experience are definitely important, you want staff members who treat the residents well.

27. **Inquire about the type of training and in-services provided for the staff members.** Basic training requirements need to be

reinforced and updated regularly, which some places voluntarily pay more attention to than others.

28. **Ask about the longevity of the nursing staff's employment.** Staff members who've been at a nursing home for a while know the routines, have well-established relationships, and can usually be counted on to deliver high-quality care. The patients matter to them. What's more, they probably like being there or they would have gone elsewhere.

29. **Learn about the licensed physicians and midlevel professionals at the facility, such as the nurse practitioners and physicians' assistants.** Knowing the schedule for their regular rounds is important. Then you know when you can communicate directly with them. It's also important to learn how many of these professionals are available to the residents of the particular nursing home you're considering.

30. **Realize that new buildings, new furniture, and new equipment, while nice to look at and important for the level of function, are no substitute for experienced, caring staff.** People matter most.

COMMUNICATING WITH YOUR HEALTH-CARE GIVERS

31. **Keep in mind that the cornerstone of nursing-home care is the care plan.** An interdisciplinary effort that receives contributions from nearly all members of the staff, this written plan is compiled soon after a resident's admission. The plan is discussed at a scheduled meeting—the care-plan meeting or care conference—to which families and cognitively capable residents are

invited. Both families and patients are encouraged to provide input at that time.

32. **Be aware that the best outcomes occur for residents whose families stay intimately involved.** That means visiting frequently, interacting closely with staff members, advocating for the patient, and overseeing the patient's care in general.

33. **Recognize who works at a nursing home and know what they do.** Nursing-home staff consists of a large cast of characters, each with specific tasks and responsibilities. See the Glossary for further guidance and explanation.

34. **Expect the most frequent interaction for residents and families to be face-to-face contact with certified nursing aides (CNAs) and nurses.** Families will also communicate a great deal with nurses by telephone.

35. **Anticipate direct patient contact with a doctor, nurse practitioner, or physician's assistant regularly.** This interface should take place anywhere from several times a week to once every other month as dictated by "medical necessity" and federal regulation. Scheduling of these meetings depends on whether a resident is a skilled-nursing (short-term) patient or a custodial-care (long-term) patient.

36. **Realize that medical personnel are usually in the facility at least once a week and will see residents if necessary or indicated.** Residents and families can always get a message to medical personnel by phone or in writing through the nursing

staff. More specifically, families can ask for phone conferences or face-to-face meetings with medical personnel.

THE RIGHTS OF RESIDENTS AND FAMILIES

37. **Understand that residents have all the rights of a United States citizen.** A second layer of protection arises from the fact that nursing homes in America are highly regulated by state governments, which are overseen by the federal government.

38. **Be conscious of the fact that individual nursing homes vary** with respect to options like providing smoking or nonsmoking facilities and allowing pets on the premises. Ask about what's allowed and available.

39. **Expect the nursing home to provide you with a copy of residents' rights as regulated by law.** These rights are discussed at length in Chapter Eight and also available at the Medicare site listed in the "Consumer Resources" section of this book. Some of these residents' rights are:

- The right to be treated with dignity and respect
- The right to be informed in writing about services and fees before a resident enters the nursing home
- The right to manage one's own money or choose a trusted person to do so
- The right to privacy and to keep and use one's personal belongings and property as long as doing so doesn't interfere with the rights, health, or safety of others

- The right to be informed about one's medical condition and medications, and to see one's own doctor, including the right to refuse medications and treatments
- The right to choose one's schedule (for example, when to get up and go to sleep), activities, and other preferences
- The right to an environment that's more like a home than an institution, maximizing comfort and providing assistance to be as independent as possible

40. **Ask about the fees for each facility.** Find out the daily or monthly fees, what is included in those fees, when the fees are payable, and what extra services are available for an extra charge.

41. **Realize that three separate payment categories exist when it comes to handling the finances for staying at a nursing home:**

- Nursing-home bills (room and board, nursing services)
- Physician services
- Medications

42. **Check the facility's policy about switching payment sources if you think that Medicaid may be an option later on.** Most facilities accept Medicaid, although they may have only a limited number of beds or rooms set aside for Medicaid patients. Medicaid pays for many people's nursing-home care, but the rules differ by state.

43. **Understand that, in the United States, each state licenses its nursing homes, making them subject to that state's laws and regulations.** All or part of a nursing home may participate in Medicare and/or Medicaid. Becoming state-certified by passing

a survey (inspection) also makes them subject to federal laws and regulations.

44. Expect the nursing-home bill to be paid in the following ways:

- Medicare Part A: for skilled nursing care
- Medicare HMOs (e.g., Secure Horizons): for skilled nursing care
- Medicaid: for long-stay patient care
- Private health insurance (e.g., Aetna): for short-stay patients not yet eligible for Medicare
- U.S. Department of Veterans Affairs: for patients staying at a VA facility or other skilled-nursing facilities that have con-tracts with the VA
- Private pay or personal funds: usually for long stays
- LTC insurance for long-term stays

45. Anticipate these sources to cover physician services:
- Medicare Part B
- Medicaid
- Medicare HMOs (e.g., Secure Horizons)
- Private health insurance
- Private pay, usually for the balance of bills not paid by insurance

46. Arrange to have any medications paid by:
- Medicare D
- Medicaid
- Private insurance

47. Realize that the only time a great deal of money comes out of your pocket for nursing-home care is when you choose to pay that way. This may happen if you or a loved one chooses to stay at an exclusive nursing home and pay for it directly. Otherwise, you or your loved one will probably qualify for Medicaid, if you meet the limited resources and residency requirements.

Get more detailed, in-depth guidance about choosing a nursing home at the following website: http://www.medicare.gov/NHCompare/. Topics covered there include the following:

- Medicare's guide to choosing a nursing home
- a nursing-home checklist
- a patient's bill of rights
- helpful organization contacts
- database of nursing homes in America (with a comparison tool)
- alternatives to nursing homes

All nursing homes in the U.S. that receive Medicare and/or Medicaid funding are subject to federal regulations. The nursing-home industry is one of the most heavily regulated industries in the United States.

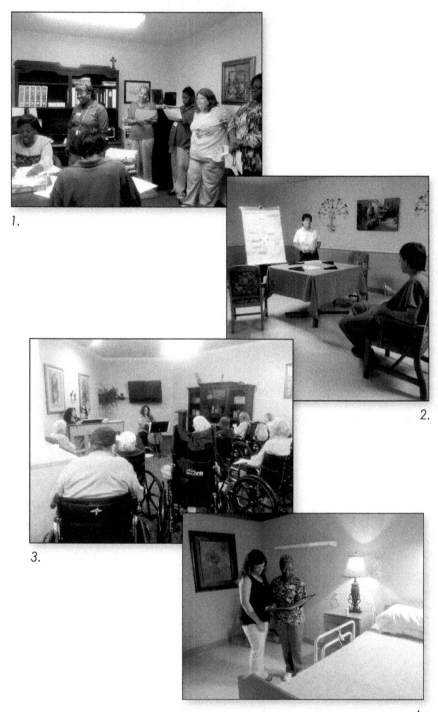

1.

2.

3.

4.

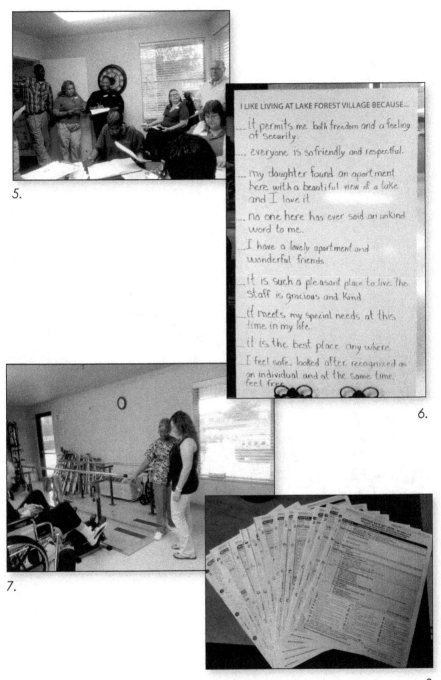

5.

I LIKE LIVING AT LAKE FOREST VILLAGE BECAUSE...

... it permits me both freedom and a feeling of security.

... everyone is so friendly and respectful.

... my daughter found an apartment here with a beautiful view of a lake and I love it

... no one here has ever said an unkind word to me.

... I have a lovely apartment and wonderful friends

... it is such a pleasant place to live. The staff is gracious and kind

... it meets my special needs at this time in my life.

... it is the best place any where.

... I feel safe, looked after, recognized as an individual and at the same time feel free

6.

7.

8.

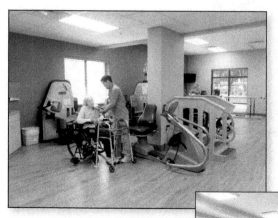

9.

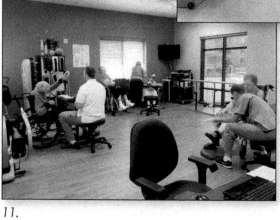

10.

11.

PHOTO CAPTIONS

1. Morning stand-up meeting

2. Continuing education for staff

3. Activites: live instrumental presentation

4. Family member touring a facility: see a room

5. Gathering for Care Plan meeting

6. What seniors want in a long-term-care facility

7. Family member touring a facility: see the gym

8. Thick MDS packet—nowadays computerized

9. One-on-one care in the rehab gym

10. Nursing home rehab gym getting big and fancy

11. One-on-one care in the gym

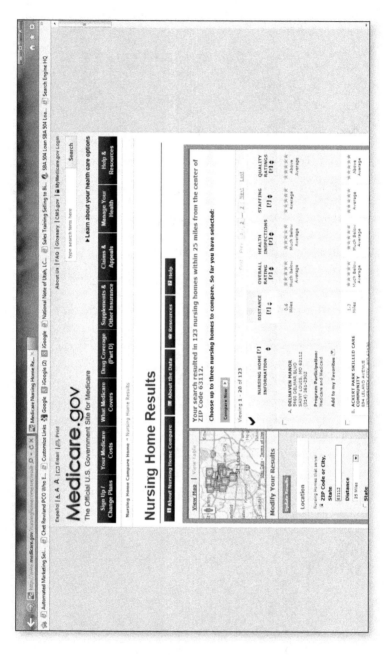

Screen shot illustrating the Five-Star Quality rating accessible on
Medicare's Nursing Home Compare website

ACKNOWLEDGMENTS

I would like the clinical team members who work with me every day in the trenches of LTC to know that I appreciate what they do for our patients and MD for Seniors. They are: Wanda Villard, NP; Dana Racinskas, NP; Kari Miley, NP; Sheila Bolanos, NP. Our experiences and conversations are now part of a book.

"Success follows management." Leading me to success at MD for Seniors and supporting me with this book project are: Amy Peabody, Clinical Practice Manager; Kristi K. C. Rawson, Chief Administrative Officer; Ariel Releford, Medical Billing Assistant.

Special thanks to my personal productivity coach Lee Milteer at Peak Performers Implementation Coaching (a Glazer-Kennedy Insider Circle program).

Thank you Dr. Gregory P. Zydiak, MD, CMD for reviewing the late-stage manuscript of this book. Your comments were invaluable.

Barbara (Barbara McNichol Editorial): You really did "add power to my pen" and your wrap-up was superb. You are super!

I also acknowledge the publishing team at Advantage Media Group:
Alison Morse, Vice President of Business Development
Denis Boyles, Editorial Director
Jenny Tripp, Project Editor

Brooke White, Senior Editor
Kim Hall, Creative and Production Director
Megan Elger, Production Assistant
Adam Witty, Founder and CEO

Thank you for carrying this project from the start to the finish line and making this book a reality.

My apologies to anyone I've forgotten to mention by name, but I still "Thank you."

RESOURCES

Abrams, Amy, MSW/MPH, CMC. "The Care Plan Conference: Making Your Voice Heard." New LifeStyles. Accessed July 7, 2012, http://www.newlifestyles.com/resources/articles/careplan.aspx.

ArcMesa Educators. "Functional Assessment: The Key to Geriatric Care in the Twenty-First Century." NursingLink. June 21, 2007. Accessed Aug. 13, 2012, http://nursinglink.monster.com/training/articles/331-functional-assess- ment---the-key-to-geriatric-care-in-the-21st-century.

Boehike, Julie. "What Are the Duties of a Nursing Home?" Livestrong.com. Sept. 9, 2009. Accessed Aug. 13, 2012, http://www.livestrong.com/article/23370-duties-nursing-home/.

Brechtelsbauer, David, MD. "We Can Dispel Long-Term Care's Bad Reputation: A Caring for the Ages." Caring for the Ages. May 2008. Accessed Aug. 13, 2012, http://www.caringfortheages.com/views/dr-b-archive/blog/we-can-dispell- long-term-care-s-bad-reputation/ddced4850aea900f2c036512e6156d9f. html.

Centers for Medicare & Medicaid Services. *Guide to Choosing a Nursing Home.* Baltimore, MD: US Dept. of Health and Human Services, Health Care Financing Administration, 2011 (1999).

Centers for Medicare & Medicaid Services. "Medicare Nursing Home Compare." Medicare Nursing Home Finder. Accessed Aug. 13, 2012, http://www.medicare.gov/NursingHomeCompare/search.aspx?bhcp=1.

Centers for Medicare & Medicaid Services. "Seniors and Medicare and Medicaid Enrollees." Medicaid. Accessed July 30, 2012, http://medicaid.gov/Medicaid-CHIP-Program-Information/By-Population/

Medicare-Medicaid-Enrollees-Dual-Eligibles/Seniors-and-Medicare-and-
Medicaid-Enrollees.html.

Centers for Medicare & Medicaid Services. "The Nursing Home Checklist." May
25, 2011. Accessed Aug. 13, 2012,
www.medicare.gov/nursing/checklist.pdf.

Chang, Louise, MD. "Nursing Home Care: Services, Costs, and More Information." WebMD. Jan. 4, 2012. Accessed Aug. 13, 2012,
http://www.webmd.com/health-insurance/nursing-home-care.

Cohen, Sylvia, Roberta DuChamp, Natalie Gordon, Wilma Greenfield, Rosalie
Kane, Carter C. Williams, Betsy Vourlekis, and Joan Levy Zlotnik. "NASW
Clinical Indicators for Social Work and Psychosocial Services in Nursing
Homes." National Association of Social Workers (NASW). Apr. 1993.
Accessed July 1, 2012,
http://socialworkers.org/practice/standards/nursing_homes.asp.

De Leon-Male, Janie, MAA, LSW, ed. "Your ADLs and IADLs." Accessed Aug.
13, 2012,
http://www.seniorcitizensguide.com/articles/southjersey/your-adls-and-
iadls.htm.

Evans, J. M., D. S. Chutka, K. C. Fleming, E. G. Tangalos, J. Vittone, and J.
H. Heathman. "Medical Care of Nursing Home Residents." *Mayo Clinic
Proceedings* 70, no. 7 (1995): 694–702.

Family Education. "Who Pays for a Nursing Home?" Excerpt from Linda Colvin
Rhodes, EdD. *The Complete Idiot's Guide to Caring for Aging Parents*. New
York: Alpha Books, 2001. Family Education. Accessed Aug. 13, 2012,
http://life.familyeducation.com/assisted-living/personal-finance/50350.
html.

Fenstemacher, Pamela Ann, and Peter S. Winn. " Nursing Facilities." *Long-term
Care Medicine: A Pocket Guide*. New York: Humana, 2011.

Ferri, Fred F., Marsha D. Fretwell, and Tom J. Wachtel. "Comprehensive
Geriatric Assessment," and Chapter Eight, "Long-Term Care." In *Practical
Guide to the Care of the Geriatric Patient*, 2nd ed. St. Louis: Mosby, 1997.

Functional Assessment - "The Key to Geriatric Care in the 21st Century." NursingLink. Ed. ArcMesa Educators. 21 June 2007. Web. 13 Aug. 2012. http://nursinglink.monster.com/training/articles/331-functional-assess-ment---the-key-to-geriatric-care-in-the-21st-century.

Funtrivia. "Nursing Home Resident's Rights." Quiz. Funtrivia. Accessed Aug. 14, 2012, http://www.funtrivia.com/en/subtopics/Nursing-Home-Residents-Rights-48451.html.

Ham, Richard J., and Philip D. Sloane. "Nursing Home Care." In *Primary Care Geriatrics: A Case-Based Approach*, 2nd ed. St. Louis: Mosby Year Book, 1992.

High, Kevin P., Suzanne F. Bradley, Stefan Gravenstein, David R. Mehr, Vincent J. Quagliarello, Chesley Richards, and Thomas T. Yoshikawa. "Clinical Practice Guideline for the Evaluation of Fever and Infection in Older Adult Residents of Long-Term Care Facilities: 2008 Update by the Infectious Diseases Society of America." *Clinical Infectious Diseases* 48.2 (2009): 149-71.

Kantor, Bonnie. "The New Nursing Home Resident's First 48 Hours." Caring for the Ages. July 1, 2010. Accessed June 18, 2012, http://www.caringfortheages.com.

Kessler, Chip. *Choices for Care*. Workbook Study Guide.

MacLean, Duncan, MD. "The Real Truth about Nursing Homes." Caring for the Ages. July 2007. Accessed Aug. 13, 2012, http://www.caringfortheages.com/views/board-room/blog/the-real-truth-about-nursing-homes/ed3c3fbf3d8b20cb00456530475a6b2d.html.

McCullough, Dennis M. *My Mother, Your Mother: Embracing "slow Medicine" - the Compassionate Approach to Caring for Your Aging Loved Ones*. New York: HarperCollins, 2009.

Nursing Home Residents Profile. Accessed June 17, 2012, http://www.amda.com/about/ltcfacts.cfm.

"Paying for Nursing Homes: Skilled Nursing Facilities." SkilledNursingFacilities. Accessed July 29, 2012, http://www.skillednursingfacilities.org/blog/category/paying-for-nursing-homes/.

Pratt, John R. "Long-Term Care Today: Turbulent Times." In *Long-term Care: Managing across the Continuum*, 3rd ed. Sudbury, MA: Jones and Bartlett, 2010.

"Residents' Rights:An Overview." NCCNHR, 27 Mar. 2007. Web.

Rhodes, Linda Colvin, Ed.D. "The Complete Idiot's Guide to Caring for Aging Parents." 2001. Paying for a Nursing Home. Web. 13 Aug. 2012, http://life.familyeducation.com/assisted-living/personal-finance/50350.html.

Saison, Joanna, MA, Doug Russell, LCSW, and Monica White, PhD. "A Guide to Nursing Homes: Skilled Nursing Facilities and Convalescent Homes." May 2012. Accessed Aug. 13, 2012, http://www.helpguide.org/elder/nursing_homes_skilled_nursing_facilities.htm.

Shook, Loren, and Stephen Winner. *The Silverado Story: A Memory-care Culture Where Love Is Greater than Fear*. Irvine, CA: AJC, 2010.

Smith, S. E. "What Is a Speech Therapist?" Ed. Bronwyn Harris. Copyright Conjecture Corporation, 2003–2012. WiseGeek. Accessed Aug. 13, 2012, http://www.wisegeek.com/what-is-a-speech-therapist.htm.

Tuggle, Mark. "Morning Meeting Makeover." Nursing Home Pro. Jan. 22, 2010. Accessed Aug. 13, 2012, http://www.nursinghomepro.com/184/morning-meeting-makeover.

Winakur, Jerald, MD. "What Are We Going to Do with Dad?" *Health Affairs* 24, no. 4 (2005): 1064–1072.

"What to Do When They Bash Your Nursing Home." Caring for the Ages. July 2010. Accessed Aug. 13, 2012, http://www.caringfortheages.com/views/meditations-on-geriatric-medicine/blog/what-to-do-when-they-bash-your-nursing-home/3116b9844ab7cf17cb5e91bbf5e38498.html.

Winn, Peter, MD, CMD, and Bonnie Wirfs, MD, CMD. "Overview of Long Term Care." Lecture presented at *AMDA Core Curriculum on Medical Direction in Long-Term Care*, Chattanoogan Hotel and Conference Center, Chattanooga, TN, June 10, 2007.

Wright, Jennifer S. "CNA Nursing Home Duties." EHow. Aug. 13, 2009. Accessed July 7, 2012, http://www.ehow.com/facts_5300939_cna-nursing-home-duties.html.

Yudt, Allison, ed. "Facts about the Five-Star Nursing Home Quality Rating System." Dec. 2, 2008. Accessed Aug. 13, 2012, http://www.adrc-tae.org.

Zydiak, Gregory P., MD CMD. *Long-Term Care Practice Manual - An Introductory Guide to the Practice of Long-Term Care Medicine*. Premier Edition. 2008.

ABBREVIATIONS

ADL – activities of daily living

ADON – assistant director of nursing

AL – assisted living

ALF – assisted-living facility

AuD – doctor of audiology

CNA – certified nurses' assistant

DDS – doctor of dental surgery

DO – doctor of osteopathy

DON – director of nursing

DPM – doctor of podiatric medicine

HHA – home-health agency

IADL – instrumental/intellectual activities of daily living

IDT – interdisciplinary team

LMSW – licensed master social worker

LPN – licensed practical nurse

LTAC – long-term acute care

LTC – long-term care

LTCF – long-term-care facility

LVN – licensed vocational nurse

MCC – memory-care center

MD – doctor of medicine

NF – nursing facility

NH – nursing home

NP – nurse practitioner

OD – doctor of optometry

OT – occupational therapist

PA – physician's assistant

PharmD – doctor of pharmacy

PM&R – physical medicine and rehabilitation doctor

PT – physical therapist

RD – registered dietician

SNF – skilled-nursing facility

ST – speech therapist

SW – social worker

Dr. Pobee has been, or still is, affiliated with the following facilities and organizations:

The Health Group
9101 LBJ Frwy., Ste. 710, Dallas, TX 75243
tel. 972-792-5700
www.thehealthgroup.org

American Medical Directors Assoc (AMDA)
11000 Broken Land Pkwy, Ste. 400
Columbia, MD 21044
tel. 410-740-9743

American Academy of Home Care Physicians (AAHCP)
PO Box 1037
Edgewood, MD 21040
tel. 410-676-7966

American Geriatrics Society (AGS)
40 Fulton St., 18th Floor
New York, NY 10038
tel. 212-308-1414

Texas Medical Directors Assoc (TMDA)
State Chapter of AMDA

Heritage Place Mesquite Nursing Home
825 W. Kearny St., Mesquite, TX 75149
tel. 972-288-7668

Willow Bend Nursing Home
2231 US Highway 80 East, Mesquite, TX 75150
tel. 972-279-3601
www.willowbendcare.com

The Meadows Health and Rehab Center
8383 Meadow Rd., Dallas, TX 75231
tel. 214-239-6000
www.SavaSC.com

Senior Care Beltline
106 N. Beltline Rd., Garland, TX 75040
tel. 972-495-7700
www.seniorcarecentersltc.com

Winters Park Nursing and Rehabilitation
3737 N. Garland Ave., Garland, TX 75040
tel. 972-495-7000
www.trisunhealthcare.com

Legend Healthcare and Rehab. Center
900 Westpark Way, Euless, TX 76040
tel. 817-545-4071
www.legendhc.com

Hurst Plaza Nursing and Rehabilitation
215 E. Plaza Blvd., Hurst, TX 76053
tel. 817-282-6777

Bishop Davies Nursing Center
2712 Hurstview Dr., Hurst, TX 76054
tel. 817-281-6707
www.bishopdaviescenter.com

Life Care Center of Haltom
2936 Markum Dr., Fort Worth, TX 76117
tel. 817-831-0545

The Carlyle at Stonebridge Park
175 Stonebridge Ln., Southlake, TX 76092
tel. 817-431-5778
www.cantexsc.com/Carlyle.php

The Harrison at Heritage
4600 Heritage Trace Pkwy, Fort Worth, TX 76244
tel. 817-741-9360
www.cantexsc.com/Harrison.php

Lake Forest Good Samaritan Village
3901 Montecito Dr., Denton, TX 76210
tel. 940-891-6443,
www.good-sam.com

The Vintage Healthcare Center
205 N. Bonnie Brae, Denton, TX 76201
tel. 940-384-1500
www.seniorcarecentersltc.com

Denton Good Samaritan Village
2500 Hinkel Dr., Denton, TX 76201
tel. 940-383-2651
www.good-sam.com

Senior Care Health and Rehab. Center, Denton
2244 Brinker Rd., Denton, TX 76208
tel. 940-320-6300
www.seniorcarecentersltc.com

Silverado Senior Living Valley Ranch
8855 W. Valley Ranch Pkwy., Irving, TX 75063
tel. 972-831-8200
www.silveradosenior.com

Good Sam. Society N. Texas Home Health Agency
1007 Shady Oaks, Ste. 101, Denton, TX 76205,
tel. 940-591-0886
www.good-sam.com

Horizon Home Health Agency
2775 Villa Creek Dr., Dallas, TX 75234
tel. 972-241-8633
www.horizonhomehealthagency.com

Charlin Home Health
400 Chisholm Dr., Plano, TX 75075
tel. 972-424-3200
www.charlinhomehealth.com

Southeast Dallas Healthcare Center of Parkland (Geriatrics Clinic)
9202 Elam Rd., Dallas, TX 75217
tel. 214-266-1706
www.parklandhospital.com/medical_services/centers_locations.
html

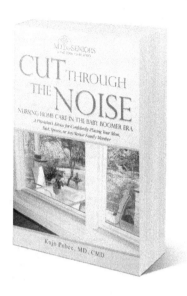

How can you use this book?

MOTIVATE

EDUCATE

THANK

INSPIRE

PROMOTE

CONNECT

Why have a custom version of *Cut through the Noise?*

- Build personal bonds with customers, prospects, employees, donors, and key constituencies
- Develop a long-lasting reminder of your event, milestone, or celebration
- Provide a keepsake that inspires change in behavior and change in lives
- Deliver the ultimate "thank you" gift that remains on coffee tables and bookshelves
- Generate the "wow" factor

Books are thoughtful gifts that provide a genuine sentiment that other promotional items cannot express. They promote employee discussions and interaction, reinforce an event's meaning or location, and they make a lasting impression. Use your book to say "Thank You" and show people that you care.